Anthony James Stewart Wright
The Longest Day - 2002
Happy Birthday,
With love from
Linda & Chris
x   x   x   x

GW00357427

# SHEPHERDS BUSH
# AND UXBRIDGE
# TRAMWAYS
## *including Ealing*

### John C Gillham
*Series editor Robert J Harley*

MP Middleton Press

# FEATURES IN LONDON TRAMWAY CLASSICS

| Rolling Stock | Title |
|---|---|
| A class. LCC | **Southwark and Deptford** |
| A type MET | **Waltham Cross and Edmonton** |
| Alexandra Palace Elec. Rly. | **Enfield and Wood Green** |
| B class. LCC/Bexley | **Greenwich and Dartford** |
| B type MET | **Stamford Hill** |
| Barking cars | **Ilford and Barking** |
| Bexley cars | **Greenwich and Dartford** |
| Bluebird. LCC car 1 | **Camberwell and West Norwood** |
| C class. LCC | **Victoria and Lambeth** |
| Cable cars | **Clapham and Streatham** |
| Croydon cars | **Croydon's Tramways** |
| C type MET/LT | **Barnet and Finchley** |
| D class. LCC | **Wandsworth and Battersea** |
| D type MET | **Edgware and Willesden** |
| Dartford cars | **Greenwich and Dartford** |
| East Ham cars | **East Ham and West Ham** |
| Erith cars | **Greenwich and Dartford** |
| E class. LCC/LT | **Aldgate and Stepney** |
| E1 class. LCC/LT | **Lewisham and Catford** |
| E1 cars 552-601. LCC/LT | **Hampstead and Highgate** |
| E1 cars 1777 -1851 LCC/LT | **Clapham and Streatham** |
| E3 class. LCC/LT | **Camberwell and West Norwood** |
| E3 class. Leyton/LT | **Walthamstow and Leyton** |
| E type MET/LT | **Enfield and Wood Green** |
| Experimental Tramcars MET/LUT/LT | **Barnet and Finchley** |
| F class. LCC | **Embankment and Waterloo** |
| F type MET | **Waltham Cross and Edmonton** |
| G class. LCC | **Embankment and Waterloo** |
| G type MET/LT | **Stamford Hill** |
| Gravesend & Northfleet cars | **North Kent** |
| H class (works). LCC/LT | **Eltham and Woolwich** |
| H type MET/LT | **Stamford Hill** |
| Horse cars. North Met./LCC | **Aldgate and Stepney** |
| HR2 class. LCC/LT | **Camberwell and W Norwood** |
| Ilford cars | **Ilford and Barking** |
| K class (works) LCC/LT | **Waltham Cross and Edmonton** |
| L class (works). LCC/LT | **Holborn and Finsbury** |
| L/1 class (works) LCC/LT | **Clapham and Streatham** |
| Leyton cars | **Walthamstow and Leyton** |
| LT car 2 | **Wandsworth and Battersea** |
| LUT car 341 | **Kingston and Wimbledon** |
| M class LCC/LT | **Greenwich and Dartford** |
| Petrol electric cars. LCC | **Southwark and Deptford** |
| SMET cars | **Croydon's Tramways** |
| S2 type LUT | **Shepherds Bush and Uxbridge** |
| T type LUT | **Kingston and Wimbledon** |
| Trailer cars LCC | **Clapham and Streatham** |
| UCC type MET/LT | **Edgware and Willesden** |
| Walthamstow cars | **Walthamstow and Leyton** |
| West Ham cars | **East Ham and West Ham** |
| Works cars MET | **Waltham Cross and Edmonton** |
| X type LUT | **Shepherds Bush and Uxbridge** |

## Miscellaneous

| | |
|---|---|
| Advertising on tramcars | **Aldgate and Stepney** |
| Conduit system | **Embankment and Waterloo** |
| Overhead wiring | **Edgware and Willesden** |
| Power supply | **Walthamstow and Leyton** |
| Request stops | **Victoria and Lambeth** |
| Section boxes | **Eltham and Woolwich** |
| Track layouts - single & loops | **Stamford Hill** |
| Track Construction and Maintenance | **Barnet and Finchley** |
| Tram tours | **Holborn and Finsbury** |

*Published December 1998*

*ISBN 1 901706 28 1*

*© Middleton Press, 1998*

*Design Deborah Goodridge*

*Published by*
*Middleton Press*
*Easebourne Lane*
*Midhurst, West Sussex*
*GU29 9AZ*
*Tel: 01730 813169*
*Fax: 01730 812601*

*Printed & bound by Biddles Ltd,*
*Guildford and Kings Lynn*

# CONTENTS

| | |
|---|---|
| Shepherds Bush | 1 |
| Acton | 22 |
| Ealing | 44 |
| Hanwell | 65 |
| Southall | 80 |
| Hayes and Hillingdon | 89 |
| Uxbridge | 99 |
| Rolling Stock | 114 |

# INTRODUCTION AND ACKNOWLEDGEMENTS

In this book we travel the main road from Shepherds Bush to Uxbridge. As well as being a very important tramway artery, it is also part of the main trunk road and one time stagecoach turnpike route from London to South Wales, via Beaconsfield, High Wycombe, Oxford, Burford, Cheltenham, Gloucester and beyond. The road as far as Uxbridge was served from 1901/04 until 1936 by the London United Electric Tramways, which also had branches off to the south from Askew Arms and from Hanwell Broadway. LUT metals were crossed by those of the LCC at Shepherds Bush Green, and were connected to those of the MET at Acton Market Place, but there were never any joint through services. Surprisingly, the inner part of this trunk road from the centre of London out as far as Shepherds Bush never had any tramways, although there were plenty of proposals which were frustrated by officialdom. The LUT lines from the Bush to Acton, from Hammersmith Broadway to Kew Bridge, and a third line linking these two, were in 1901 the very first electric street tramways in the London area.

For the photographs I am very grateful to many different people who have helped me over the past fifty years. My special thanks go to Dave Jones who has kindly loaned me valuable views from his own LUT collection, also to the late Bob Parr, who made thousands of copy negatives of old tramway photos whose origin is not known.

Timetables and other LT material are by kind permission of the London Transport Museum, Covent Garden.

Many people have helped with snippets of information, and having lived in Ealing my entire life, I have personal memories of the LUT tramways, even though it is now 62 years since they were abandoned. As a child I was a passenger on the last tram on the final evening through Ealing to Hanwell Depot.

# GEOGRAPHICAL SETTING

The Shepherds Bush to Uxbridge tramway passed through seven different boroughs or urban districts on its 12.25 mile/19 kms journey. Shepherds Bush itself was a part of the large Borough of Hammersmith, on the edge of the continuous built up area of London. Acton, Ealing, Hanwell, Southall and Uxbridge were originally self contained towns on the turnpike road to South Wales. Hayes End on the tramway was an outpost of Hayes, and Hillingdon was a quiet country village. All places on the route have now been swamped by the expansion of the metropolis. This was further accelerated when on 1st April 1965 all truly "local" government disappeared with the setting up of large London Boroughs under the aegis of the Greater London Council. Until 1888 the entire route lay within the County of Middlesex. The main activity along most of the route was originally market gardening and nurseries.

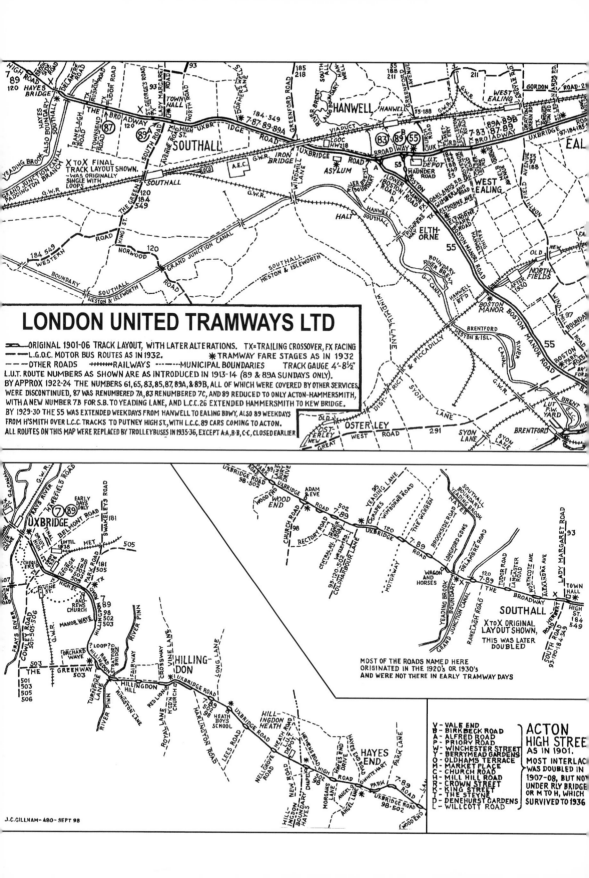

# LONDON UNITED TRAMWAYS LTD

ORIGINAL 1901-06 TRACK LAYOUT, WITH LATER ALTERATIONS. TX=TRAILING CROSSOVER, FX FACING
L.G.O.C. MOTOR BUS ROUTES AS IN 1932. ☀ TRAMWAY FARE STAGES AS IN 1932
OTHER ROADS ╫╫╫╫ RAILWAYS ┄┄ MUNICIPAL BOUNDARIES TRACK GAUGE 4'-8½'
L.U.T. ROUTE NUMBERS AS SHOWN ARE AS INTRODUCED IN 1913-14 (89 & 89A SUNDAYS ONLY).
BY APPROX 1922-24 THE NUMBERS 61,65,83,85,87,89A, & 89B, ALL OF WHICH WERE COVERED BY OTHER SERVICES,
WERE DISCONTINUED, 87 WAS RENUMBERED 7A, 83 RENUMBERED 7C, AND 89 REDUCED TO ONLY ACTON-HAMMERSMITH,
WITH A NEW NUMBER 7B FOR S.B. TO YEADING LANE, AND L.C.C.26 EXTENDED HAMMERSMITH TO KEW BRIDGE.
BY 1929-30 THE 55 WAS EXTENDED WEEKDAYS FROM HANWELL TO EALING BDWY, ALSO 89 WEEKDAYS
FROM H'SMITH OVER L.C.C. TRACKS TO PUTNEY HIGH ST, WITH L.C.C. 89 CARS COMING TO ACTON.
ALL ROUTES ON THIS MAP WERE REPLACED BY TROLLEYBUSES IN 1935-36, EXCEPT A-A, B-B, C-C, CLOSED EARLIER

MOST OF THE ROADS NAMED HERE
ORIGINATED IN THE 1920's OR 1930's
AND WERE NOT THERE IN EARLY TRAMWAY DAYS

X to X ORIGINAL
LAYOUT SHOWN,
THIS WAS LATER
DOUBLED

V - VALE END
B - BIRKBECK ROAD
A - ALFRED ROAD
P - PRIORY ROAD
W - WINCHESTER STREET
Y - BERRYMEAD GARDENS
O - OLDHAMS TERRACE
M - MARKET PLACE
C - CHURCH ROAD
H - MILL HILL ROAD
R - CROWN STREET
T - THE STEYNE
D - DENEHURST GARDENS
W - WILLCOTT ROAD

ACTON
HIGH STREE
AS IN 1901.
MOST INTERLAC
WAS DOUBLED IN
1907-08, BUT NOT
UNDER RLY BRIDGE
OR M TO H, WHICH
SURVIVED TO 1936

J.C. GILLHAM - 480 - SEPT 98

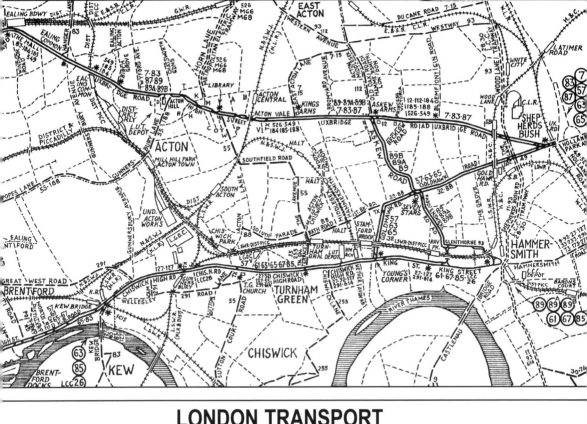

# LONDON TRANSPORT

Route diagram for 1934

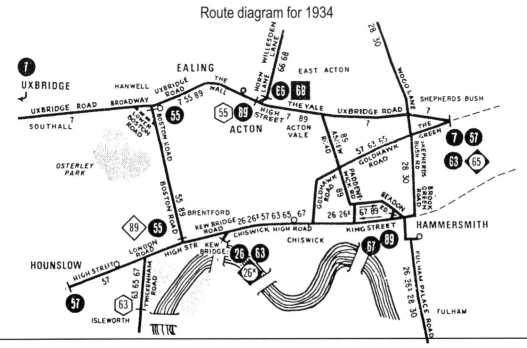

# HISTORICAL BACKGROUND

The Southall, Ealing and Shepherds Bush Tram-Railway Co Ltd was formed in 1870 with powers to make 6.9 miles/ 11 kms of horse tramway. At that time there was a half-hourly horse bus service from London to Ealing, but only twice a day thence to Uxbridge. The Great Western Railway roughly paralleled the tram route as far as Hayes, but its services were less frequent. On 1st June 1874 the SE&SB opened 1.1 miles/1.7kms of tramway from Uxbridge Road Station on the West London Railway, (described fully in the Middleton Press book - *West London Line - London Suburban Railways* series) as far as the Princess Victoria public house on the corner of Becklow Road. The route was single track with three passing loops. Sadly, that was the sum total of the SE&SB. They had failed to pay the contractor who had built the line, so service was suspended for seven months, and then the liquidator leased the operation to Charles Courtney Cramp, who reopened it on 21st September 1875. On 25th January 1878 the line was purchased by the original contractor, Reid Brothers, who extended it on 18th February 1878 a further mile to Priory Road (now Acton Lane), and the SE&SB was wound up on 4th May 1883.

A new West Metropolitan Tramways Co Ltd was formed, which purchased the tramway on 6th March 1882. An Act of 1889 authorised the double tracking of the existing route, but an intended extension from Acton to Hanwell was rejected. Financial problems arose and a receiver was appointed on 24th August 1893. He was George White, Chairman of the Bristol Tramways & Carriage Co Ltd. After failing to find a bidder at an auction on 13th August 1894, the WMT was purchased by Mr Krauss, who was acting on behalf of the Bristol company; on 20th August the new London United Tramways Co was formed. After numerous postponements the existing single track tramway with eight loops was at last relaid and doubled throughout (except under the NLR bridge at Acton) in the summer of 1895. Also the line was extended on 31st August 1895 from Priory Road to the top of Acton Hill, just beyond Gunnersbury Lane, where a large new tram depot and stables was constructed on the south side of the main road.

Further parliamentary powers were obtained and the route from Shepherds Bush to Acton Hill was electrified on 4th April 1901, and extended to Southall Town Hall on 10th July 1901. The whole section was double track. On 1st June 1904 a further extension took the rails to the far end of Uxbridge High Street at Harefield Road. This was built as single track with 23 passing loops and then double for the last three-quarters of a mile. A large tram depot was erected in Hanwell Broadway and a smaller one at Hillingdon Heath. On 4th April 1901 the LUT also electrified the horse tramway (originally opened on 18th March 1882) from Shepherds Bush, via Goldhawk Road, to Youngs Corner at Chiswick. A new branch tramway from the county boundary at Askew Arms, via Askew Road and Paddenswick Road, to Hammersmith Broadway opened on 1st June 1901. Finally a route from Hanwell Broadway, via both Upper and Lower Boston Road, to Brentford Half Acre saw service from 26th May 1906.

Route numbers were allocated to all LUT services in 1913-14, these being odd numbers from 55 to 89, except 59 and 79. Even numbers were allocated to the MET services. This was the result of financial control of both the London United and the Metropolitan Electric being acquired on 1st January 1913 by the London and Suburban Traction Co Ltd. The Uxbridge Road service and its short workings became 83, 87 and 89, but in about 1923 these were renumbered 7, 7A, 7B and 7C.

The very short line in Lower Boston Road was never used much and was abandoned in about 1910. All the other routes passed on 1st July 1933 to the control of London Transport, who shortly formulated a policy of trolleybus replacement of tramway services. Goldhawk Road was converted on 27th October 1935, Askew Arms to Hammersmith on 5th April 1936, the main trunk Uxbridge route on 15th November 1936, and Boston Road to Brentford on 13th December 1936. The Boston Road tram service had been extended beyond Hanwell to Ealing Broadway since 9th November 1928, and this continued for the four weeks from 15th November to 12th December 1936 along this part of the otherwise abandoned main Uxbridge route. The replacing trolleybus routes 607 and 655 ran for the last time on 8th November 1960 when they were in turn replaced by diesel buses.

# SHEPHERDS BUSH

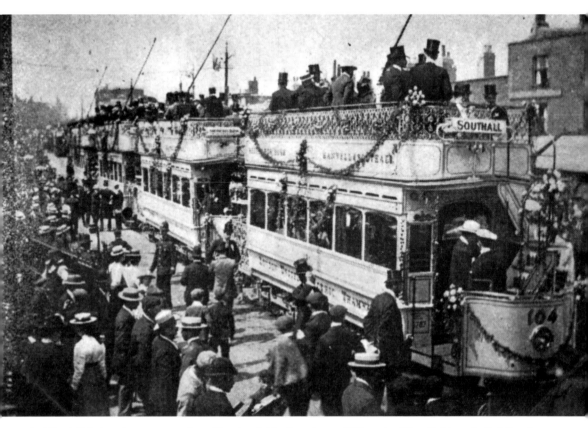

1. The LUT electric tramways from Shepherds Bush to Acton Hill, and to Kew Bridge via Goldhawk Road, had been ready for nearly a year, but a fierce battle was being fought with officialdom. The trouble was mainly with the Kew Observatory authorities, who insisted that return electric currents from tramrails would damage their sensitive instruments. The LUT was desperate to get the trams running in time for the Easter weekend crowds. Permission was granted with a day to spare! In a huge, hectic rush all the electric cars started running on Maunday Thursday, 4th April 1901. There was no time to arrange a grand opening ceremony, and this had to wait until 10th July, as shown in this picture at the Bush looking west. (LUT)

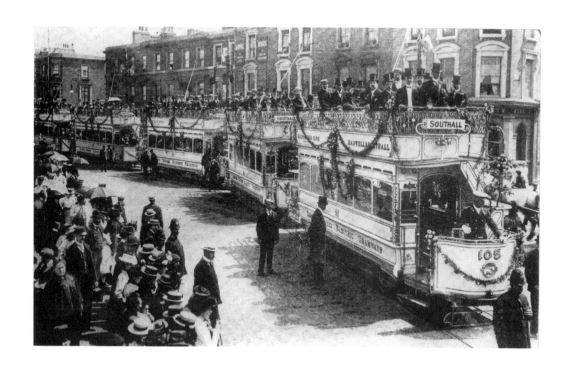

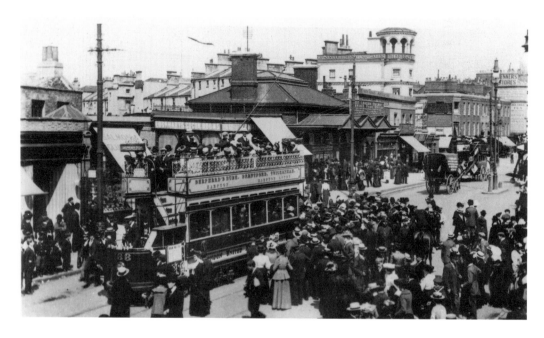

2. Cars 101 to 109 were gaily decorated with flowers and bunting for the opening ceremony. The trams were packed solid with 450 important people from the municipal, parliamentary, tramway, electrical, industrial and commercial spheres. Here we see the procession ready to start; even the driver is wearing white gloves. The party went to Southall and back, then finished up in Chiswick Depot for a gigantic banquet. In this picture, looking east, the two trams in the foreground are at the end of Uxbridge Road, and those round the corner are in the beginning of Holland Park Avenue. All the buildings visible here were demolished in about 1970-80, and replaced by large retail shops. (LUT)

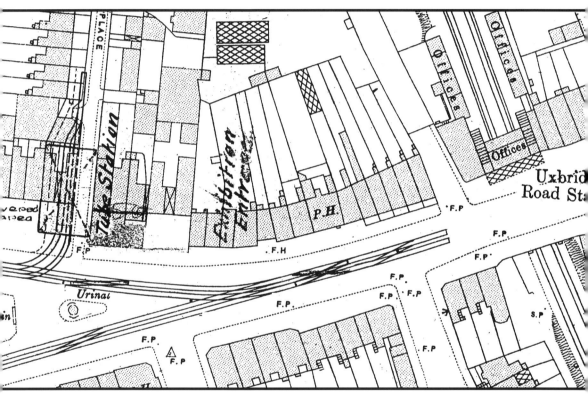

The 1895 edition at 50ins to 1 mile has the WLR on the right. For full details of this unusual route, see *West London Line* (Middleton Press). The plan includes details of the 1907 proposals for an off-street terminal. Unfortunately this scheme never came to frutition.

3. The tram tracks in Uxbridge Road and Goldhawk Road joined together and continued a short distance to end outside Uxbridge Road Station on the West London Railway, whose surface buildings we see in the centre of this picture. A large crowd is trying to squeeze on to car 168 for a trip to Hampton Court on August Bank Holiday, 3rd August 1903. In modern times every trace of the WLR station and the surrounding buildings has been destroyed and the whole area has been cleared for a new roundabout and dual carriageway road leading north to Western Avenue. (Pamlin Prints)

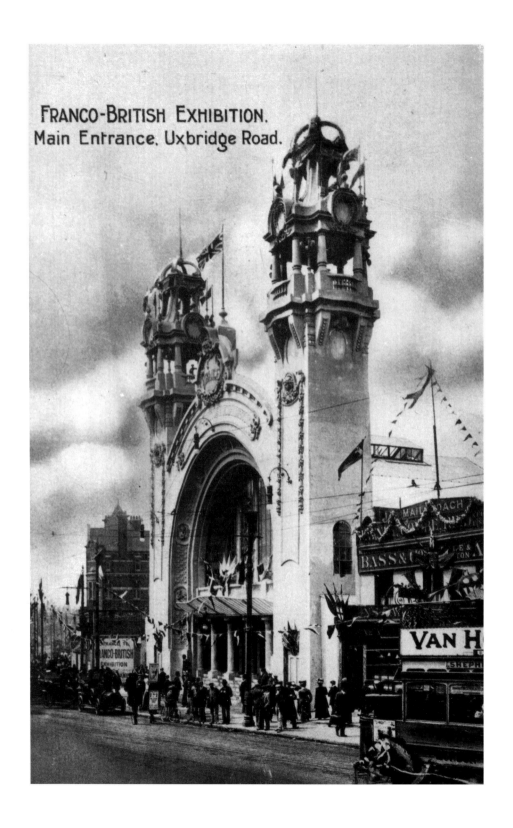

FRANCO-BRITISH EXHIBITION.
Main Entrance, Uxbridge Road.

←——

4.　The Franco-British Exhibition was held at Shepherds Bush in the summer of 1908. Most of the show was in an area which is bounded today by Wood Lane, Western Avenue, Bloemfontein Road and the Queens Park Rangers football ground. The main entrance lay between the WLR station and the junction of the two LUT routes, access being by a temporary ornamental bridge over Wood Lane. Here we see the main entrance in all its glory with part of an LUT tramcar on the right. This structure still exists, except that the tops of the two towers have long since vanished. The Mail Coach public house on the right was later demolished and replaced by a new building on the same site with the same name. (J.W.Stuchlik)

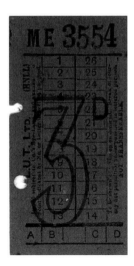

5.　LUT car 120, of the 101-150 type, which were at first painted white and always worked on the Uxbridge Road services, but did not survive as long as other LUT types, is standing outside Shepherds Bush Station of the Central London Railway. We are looking east, with Goldhawk Road just off to the right and the start of Holland Park Avenue visible in the distance.　Throughout tramway operation the terminus remained outside the CLR station, and the LUT gave great publicity to the fact that they connected so closely, with joint through booking tickets. The trolleybuses also set down here, although passengers were only picked up further away in Goldhawk Road. For many years now the replacing buses have only run as far as Caxton Road, leaving crowds of through passengers a long walk to the station.　(Commercial Postcard)

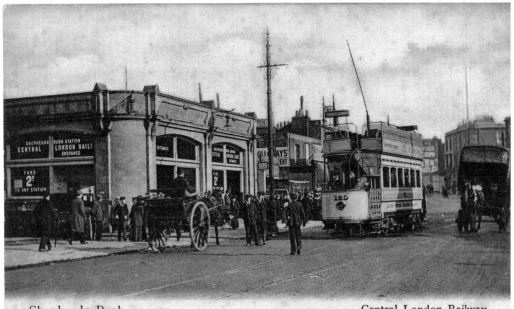

Shepherds Bush.　　　　　　　　　　　　　　　　　Central London Railway.

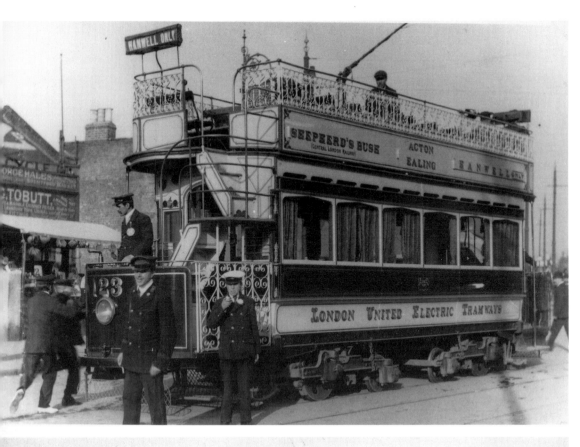

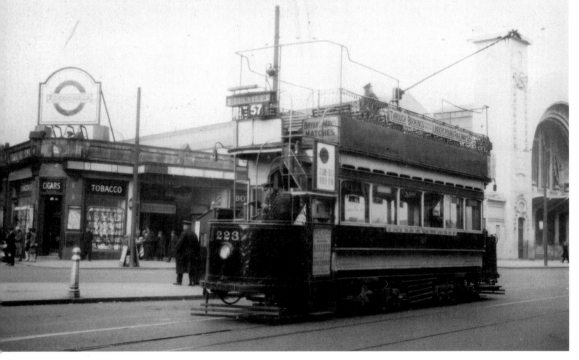

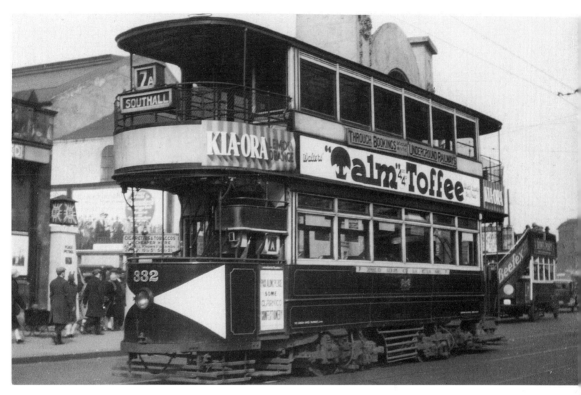

6.  Car 123 stands at the terminus in about 1920. Note the detachable route boards on the upper deck sides which inform us HANWELL ONLY instead of Southall or Uxbridge. Note also the unusual double right angle staircase, which was standard to all the first 340 LUT trams (only the last 46 did not have them) - this is known as a "Robinson staircase" after the General Manager, Sir James Clifton Robinson.  (Dave Jones Coll.)

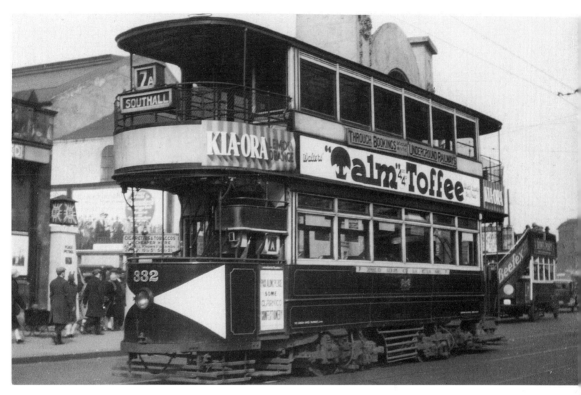

7.    Car 223 stands at the Goldhawk Road terminus in 1928. The Uxbridge Road terminus alongside is empty at this moment. The CLR station has had some minor alterations since it was built in 1900. Note the large board along the top of the tram - THROUGH BOOKINGS WITH THE UNDERGROUND RAILWAYS. In 1998 this scene is dominated by a huge artificial advertising bridge across both main roads. (G.N.Southerden)

8.    The end of the CLR station is just visible on the extreme left of car 332. Some of the T type trams, 301-340, had these white triangles painted on the dash to remind drivers of motor vehicles that they had eight wheel brakes and had been recently fitted with more powerful motors. The K type bus of the London General Omnibus Co Ltd reminds us that by 1930 there were six different bus routes from various parts of LUT territory to the centre of London. These competed with the LUT/CLR interchange, even though tram, tube and bus companies were under the same overall ownership.  (G.N.Southerden)

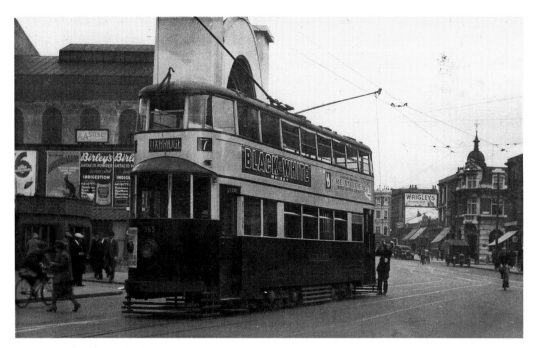

9. The luxurious new UCC or Feltham type tram of 1931 was used for six years on the Uxbridge route, before being sent south to Streatham Depot. This view shows that the junction between the Uxbridge Road and Goldhawk Road tracks was still in situ in 1932, although not normally used. All the buildings on the right of this picture have been demolished in recent years. (G.N.Southerden)

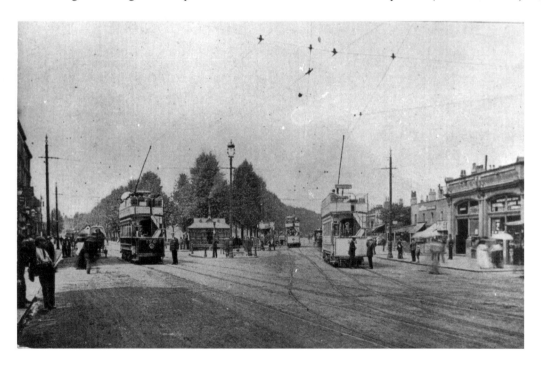

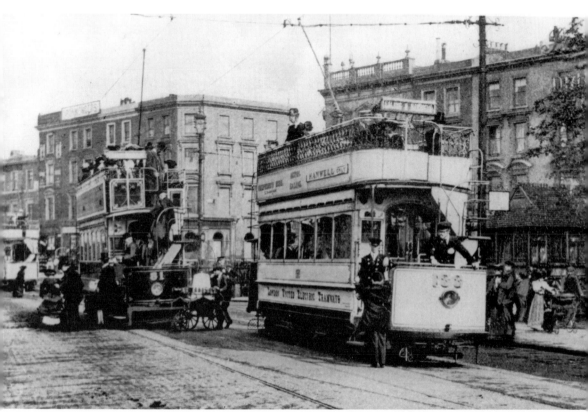

11. Trams 81 and 133 stand at the Uxbridge Road terminus. Note the higher side panels and square corners of the top deck of type Z on the left, and the lower panels and rounded corners of type X on the right. Both originally had destination boards, but now have roller blind boxes instead - in later life they reverted to boards. An old fashioned milkman with his churn on a wheelbarrow is crossing the road, and the cabmen's shelter is on the right.
(Commercial Postcard)

10. We now direct our attention towards the west, with Goldhawk Road on the left and Uxbridge Road on the right. In the centre is Shepherds Bush Green, a public open space since 1872, with the cabmen's shelter visible and a horse drinking trough in front of it. The tram on the left is painted dark blue, whilst the one on the right is white. Bodywork of both is very similar, but trucks and equipment are of different types. The CLR station is on the right; the buildings beyond were demolished in about 1904-06, and this picture was published in 1904.   (A.J.Peake)

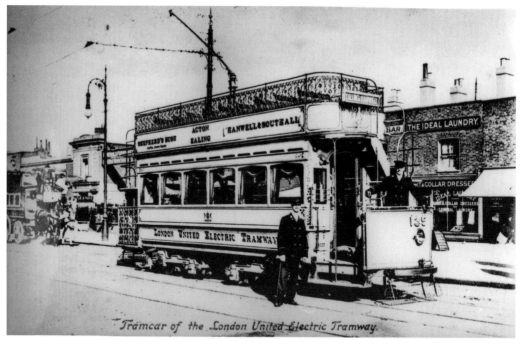

*Tramcar of the London United Electric Tramway.*

12. Car 135, with G.F.Milnes bodywork, McGuire trucks, and Westinghouse motors and controllers, stands at the terminus in the first few years. Note the horse bus behind the tram. The CLR station is just off the edge of the picture to the right. All the buildings visible were demolished in 1904-06 and replaced by a parade of four storey shops of attractive appearance.   (Commercial Postcard)

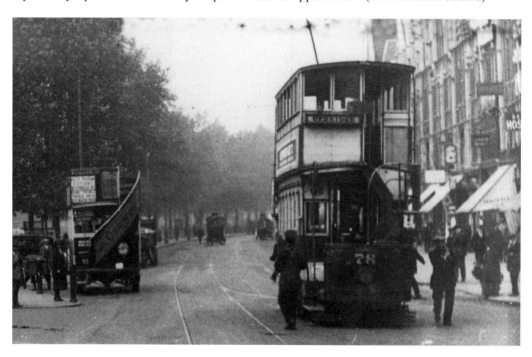

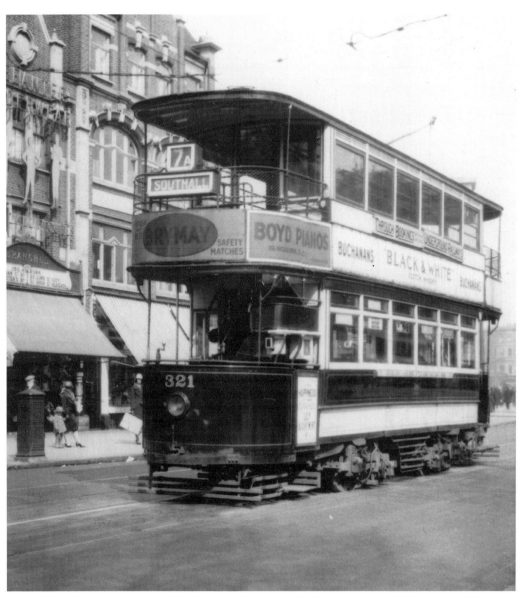

13. Sixty-six of the first hundred cars were fitted with uncanopied top covers in 1909-10, thus becoming (when class letters were allocated in 1913) type Y. Here is one of them on the north side of Shepherds Bush Green. The parade of tall buildings on the right was built in about 1907-08. The LGOC K type motor bus has just reached its terminus here, after coming all the way from Dulwich via Oxford Circus on route 12. (George Robbins Coll.)

14. Unlike the first 300 cars, the 40 which were later known as type T had covered tops and end canopies when new. They were built in 1906 and worked for a year or two in the Kingston area, but following complaints about the low power of the 1-100 and 101-150 types on the Shepherds Bush routes, ten of these 301-340 cars were transferred in 1907-08 to the Hounslow route and thirty to the Uxbridge Road route, where they all remained until 1936. (G.N.Southerden)

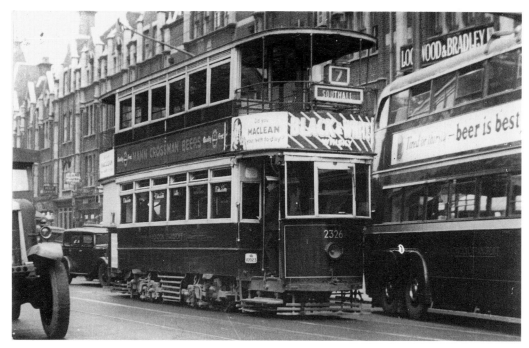

15.  Pictured is type T car 310 in 1936, after it had been acquired and renumbered by London Transport. Some of this type were fitted with drivers' windscreens in about 1931. The location is the same as the previous picture, but looking in the other direction. The trolleybus is on route 657 which replaced the Goldhawk Road to Hounslow tram service. The lorry on the left is a Leyland, then about ten years old. Being almost at the terminus, the tram's destination blind has already been changed.  (M.J.O'Connor)

16.  Car 113 is depicted on the north side of Shepherds Bush Green, with Aldine Street on the right and Wood Lane beyond. All the buildings in this picture still survive unaltered. (Commercial Postcard)

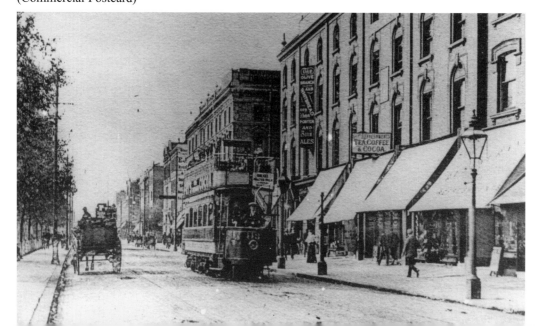

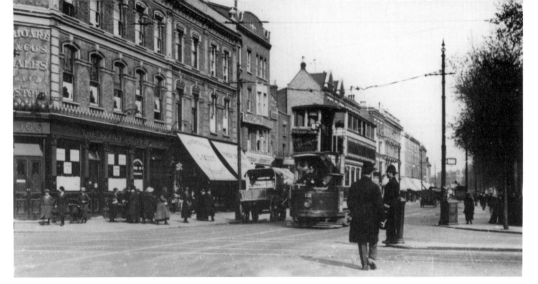

17.  Here we are looking eastwards along the north side of Shepherds Bush Green, with car 13 of type Y. In the foreground the tracks of the London County Council Tramways cross at right angles, and they did likewise across Goldhawk Road on the far side of the Green, but there was no junction or pointwork at either crossing. This LCC route ran from Hammersmith to Harlesden via Wood Lane, and is partly covered in companion volume *Edgware and Willesden Tramways*. It opened on 30th May 1908 and was the second complete LCC route to employ overhead trolley instead of the conduit system. The LUT car displays route number 87, which makes it 1914 or slightly later. (Commercial Postcard)

18.  We now advance along Wood Lane to marvel at the splendour of the Franco-British Exhibition opened in May 1908, just a few days before the LCC tramway. The bridge on the right, despite being such an imposing structure, was only temporary, and led through to the Uxbridge Road entrance (see picture 4). An LCC E class tram can just be seen underneath the bridge. The motor bus is a Vanguard, probably on a Milnes-Daimler chassis, shortly before Vanguard was amalgamated with the LGOC. (Commercial Postcard)

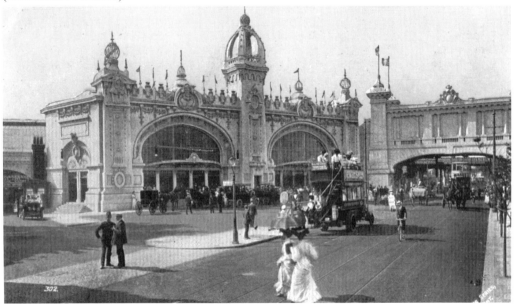

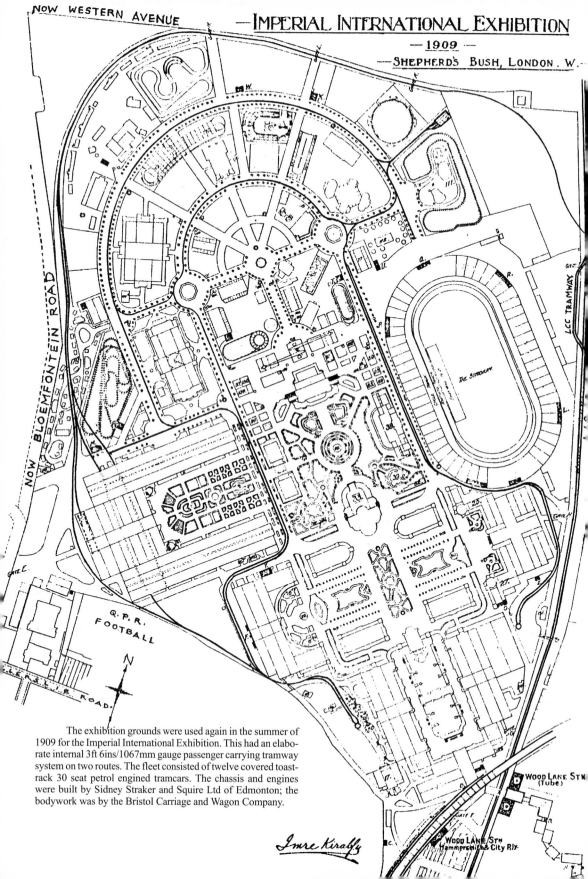

# IMPERIAL INTERNATIONAL EXHIBITION
## — 1909 —
### — SHEPHERD'S BUSH, LONDON . W.

NOW WESTERN AVENUE

NOW BLOEMFONTEIN ROAD

LCC TRAMWAY

THE STADIUM

Q.P.R. FOOTBALL

LESLIE ROAD

N

WOOD LANE STN (Tube)

WOOD LANE STN Hammersmith & City Rly.

The exhibition grounds were used again in the summer of 1909 for the Imperial International Exhibition. This had an elaborate internal 3ft 6ins/1067mm gauge passenger carrying tramway system on two routes. The fleet consisted of twelve covered toast-rack 30 seat petrol engined tramcars. The chassis and engines were built by Sidney Straker and Squire Ltd of Edmonton; the bodywork was by the Bristol Carriage and Wagon Company.

*Imre Kiralfy*

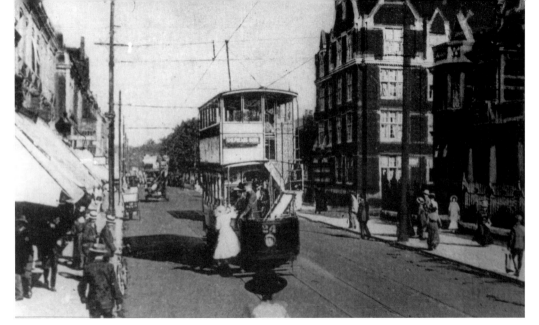

19.  We look east in Uxbridge Road on the Acton side of Wood Lane to observe another Y type tram. The camera is almost underneath the Hammersmith & City Railway bridge. The building on the extreme right is Shepherds Bush Public Library, which was built in 1895 on a site which in 1874 had been partly occupied by the depot and stables of the original SE&SB tramway. All the buildings in this picture still survive.  (Commercial Postcard)

20.  T type car 336 is seen in about 1920, together with an LGOC bus B1997 on route 17 from London Bridge Station to Ealing Broadway. The H&C railway bridge can just be seen in the far distance. St.Stephen's Church is on the corner of Coverdale Road; all the houses on the right were built in 1874, and all still survive.  (A.D.Packer)

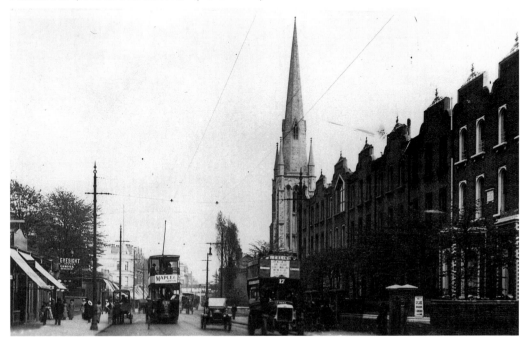

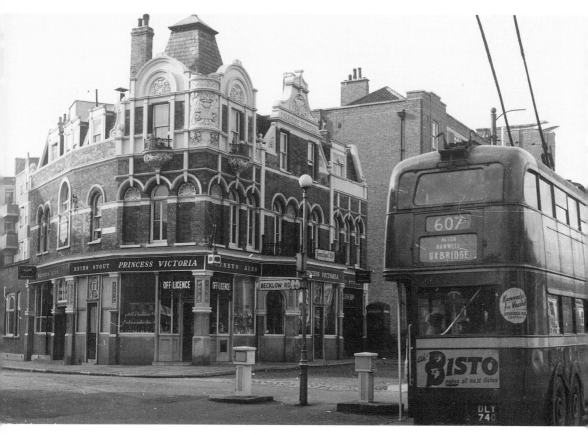

21. The Princess Victoria Hotel on the corner of Becklow Road was the terminus of the original SE&SB horse tramway, until the 1878 extension to Priory Road. The cobble stoned yard outside the Princess Victoria was also the terminus of several motor bus routes in the first 30 years of the present century. This view was taken in 1960.   (John Gillham)

23.   The Askew Arms Hotel, seen on the right of the picture, was an important landmark in LUT history. It was a main fare stage and it stood on the county boundary which marked the point of change of ownership of the tramway. For 34 years the LCC felt it should own all the tramways inside the County of London, and the LUT lines from Shepherds Bush to Askew Arms and along Goldhawk Road and King Street, Hammersmith were the last sections to be acquired. After some stout resistance they were compulsorily purchased by the LCC on 2nd May 1922. However, the LUT was still allowed to operate through services. This picture of car 335 coming from the Bush probably dates to just before 1913.   (Commercial Postcard)

# ACTON

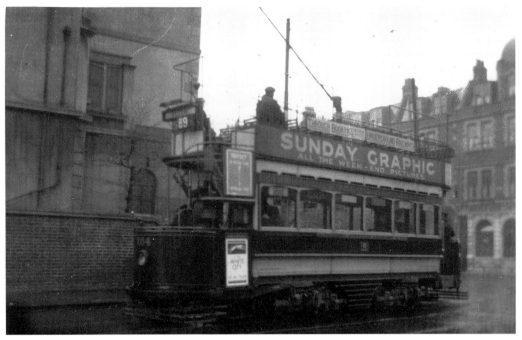

22. Type W car 164 emerges from Askew Road in about 1930-32, and is about to turn left into Uxbridge Road, on its journey from Hammersmith Broadway to Acton High Street. The county boundary between London and Middlesex, and between the Boroughs of Hammersmith and Acton was at this point. One of the factors which delayed the opening of the LUT tramway by about a year in 1900-01 was the insistence of the LCC that the tramway in its territory, amounting to just over a mile in length, should be constructed on the conduit system. The LUT was adamant that it must be overhead wires. A fierce battle raged, but the LUT won in the end.   (W.Noel Jackson)

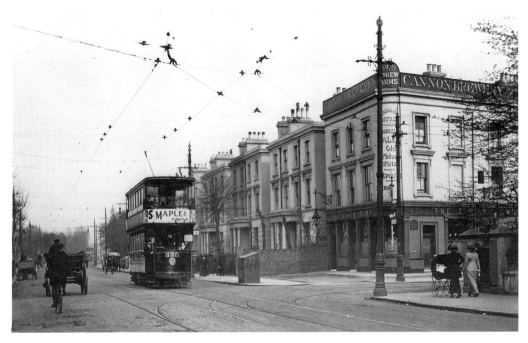

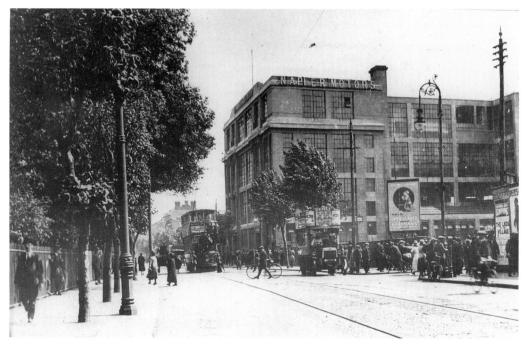

24. Further along Uxbridge Road in Acton Vale a tram is passing the factory of D.Napier & Sons Ltd, a manufacturer of motor cars and lorries, also aero engines in the 1914-18 war. It seems to be knocking off time and crowds of workers are trying to board the tram and the competing General bus.  (Commercial Postcard)

25.  There was a section of interlaced track where the LUT tramway passed under the railway from Willesden Junction to Richmond. This configuration remained to the end, but several other interlaced sections through Acton were later doubled. Soon after the trams were abandoned in 1936, a new and much wider bridge was substituted. The Napier factory can be seen in the distance behind one of the two T type trams.   (B.J.Cross Coll.)

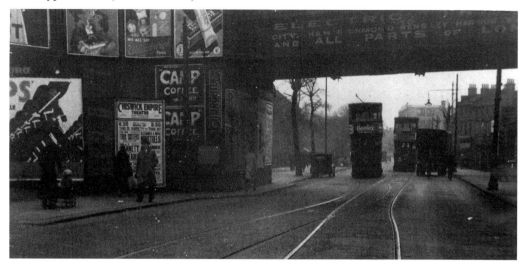

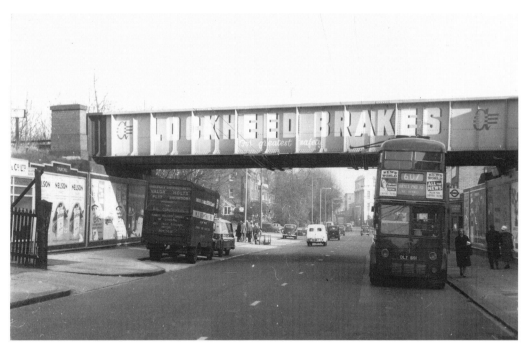

26. This picture, taken on 7th November 1960, shows the new and wider bridge. Note that both bridges had only just enough head clearance for the trolley poles. (John Gillham)

27. We come a little further west to the corner of Alfred Road. The section of interlaced track here was doubled at a fairly early date. All the buildings still exist, but the tall one on the extreme left was later replaced by a Granada Cinema, which is now a Bingo Hall. (Commercial Postcard)

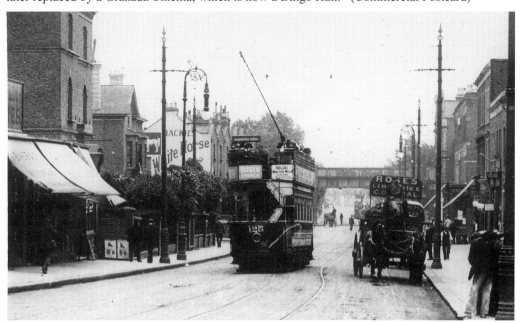

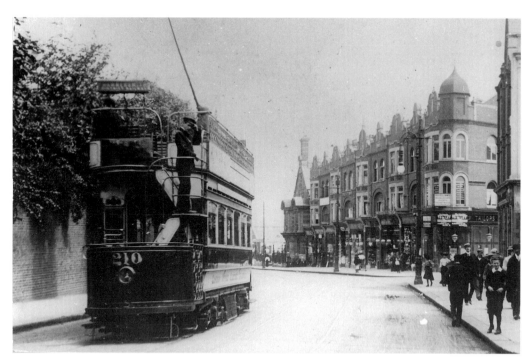

28. Looking east from the centre of Acton in 1907, we view the High Street with Berrymead Gardens on the right, and Acton Library in the middle. Car 210 displays HAMMERSMITH DISTRICT RAILWAY on its destination blind - it will be travelling via Askew Road and Paddenswick Road. Other trams in this era displayed SHEPHERDS BUSH CENTRAL LONDON RAILWAY in lettering almost too small to read.   (Acton Public Library)

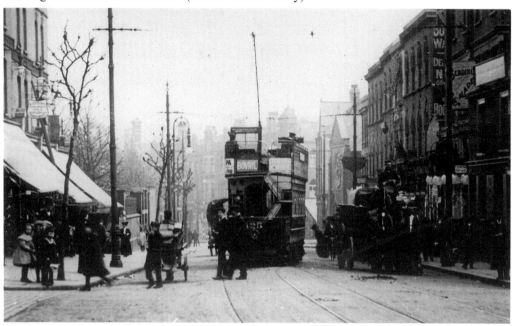

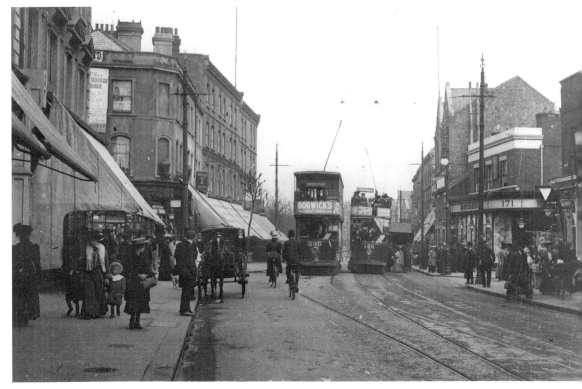

←

29.  We now find ourselves in Acton High Street, looking east from the corner of Market Place. Car 125 is about to enter a short section of single track (later doubled) outside the Roman Catholic Church.  (Commercial Postcard)

30.  Trams 335 and 148 are passing on the double track in Acton High Street, opposite Market Place on the left and Church Road to the right. Interlaced track is in the foreground and single track lies behind the trams. This piece of the High Street is still narrow in the 1990s. (R.J.Harley Coll.)

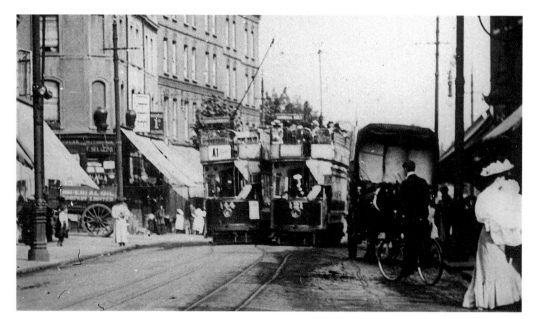

31. Cars 144 and 121 are at exactly the same spot as the previous picture, but viewed from a different angle, in both cases looking east. Note the full load of passengers on both top decks. The layout of tracks at this location allowed delivery vans to unload at the kerb. (Commercial Postcard)

32. This view was taken between 1895 and 1900 when Acton High Street had a single track horse tramway. We are looking west from Oldhams Terrace, and the Market Place for Horn Lane goes off to the right at the slight bend beyond Goddards Boot Stores. All the buildings on the right and most of those on the left still exist, but the single storey properties were replaced in 1904. (Commercial Postcard)

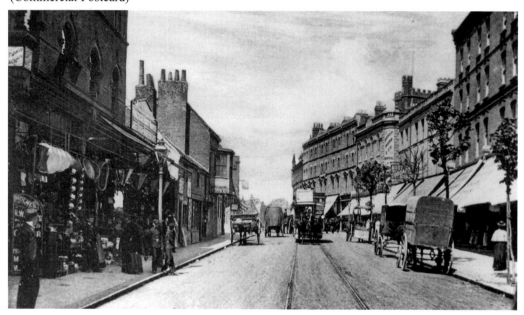

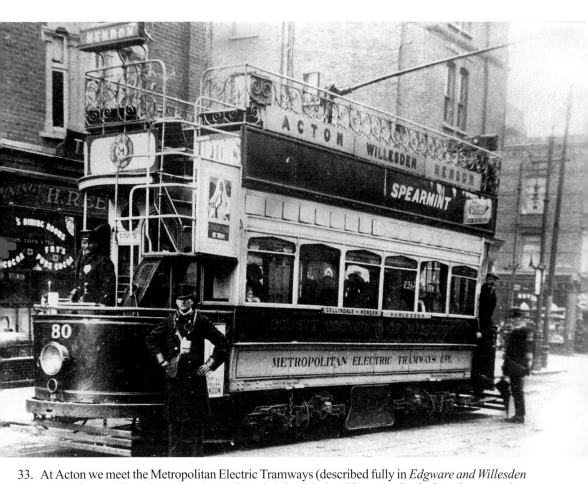

33. At Acton we meet the Metropolitan Electric Tramways (described fully in *Edgware and Willesden Tramways*) here at Horn Lane terminus where it joins Market Place. A physical track connection with LUT lines was laid in 1915, but there were never any through services. The connecting line was used in emergencies and for fleet transfers between the LUT and MET, especially for those LUT cars which needed access to Hendon Depot and its overhaul works. The Horn Lane tramway ran from 8th October 1909 to 4th July 1936 when a through trolleybus service was instituted. In 1994 King Street was closed to all traffic, and buses were diverted via a new road in the wilderness further west, thus by-passing the southern part of Horn Lane - a major nuisance for the shopkeepers and their customers!   (C.Carter)

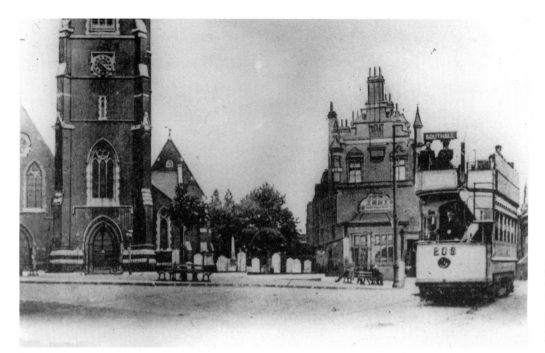

34. LUT tram 203, one of the very few type W cars which were painted white or yellow in the early days, is seen at the western end of the High Street. St.Mary's Parish Church and Barclays Bank (built in 1862) still exist, but a new church hall, with offices above, was built in the space between them in the spring of 1997. King Street goes off to the left. (Commercial Postcard)

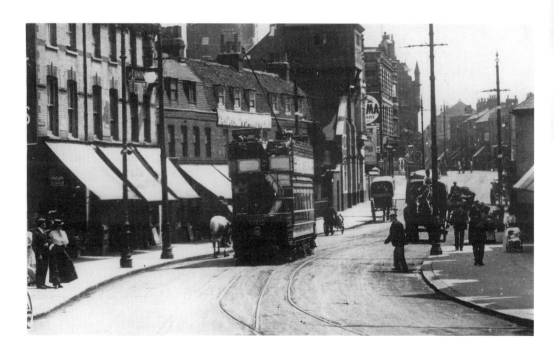

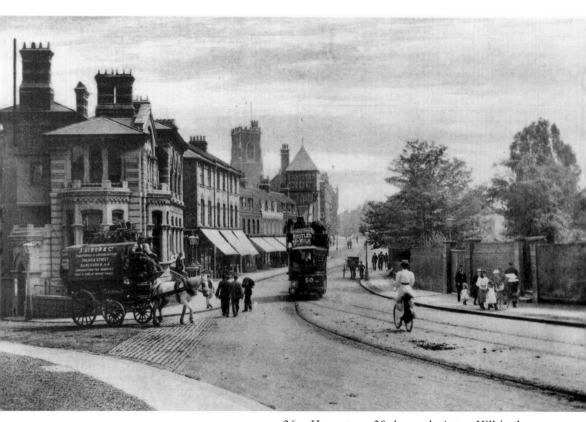

←

35. Tram 132 is here descending Acton Hill on another of the five interlaced sections which were doubled in 1907. This car was a member of type X, which were originally painted white and many of them were later repainted red. They were not used much after 1908, then they were stored and sold or scrapped in 1922-24. King Street is off to the left in the far distance. Everything in the left half of this picture was demolished in 1991-92. Steyne Road is off the bottom left corner. (Commercial Postcard)

36. Horse tram 30 descends Acton Hill in the 1895 to 1900 period, having just come off a passing loop on to single track. Nowadays a gigantic Safeway supermarket, plus its even larger car park, dominates the scene to the left of the picture. The long low building was T.Poore & Sons, Ironmongers, a family business dating back 165 years through five generations of the family. It is now banished to an obscure back street half a mile away from the nearest bus service. (Commercial Postcard)

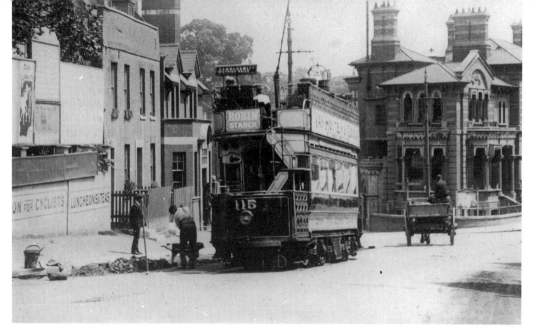

37.  We look east from near the corner of Gunnersbury Lane to observe car 115 as it descends Acton Hill. The building on the right was demolished by 1960 and the site was later used to widen Steyne Road.   (Commercial Postcard)

38.  The horse tramway through Acton was extended in 1895 from Priory Road to just beyond Gunnersbury Lane, and a new depot and stables were built at the terminus. Here we are looking west, with the depot on the left, and four of the company's staff are posing for their portrait. Springfield College was later replaced by a parade of retail shops. The tram's destination board reads rather repetitively UXBRIDGE RD STN & ACTON VIA UXBRIDGE ROAD & HIGH ST ACTON. (Middlesex County Times)

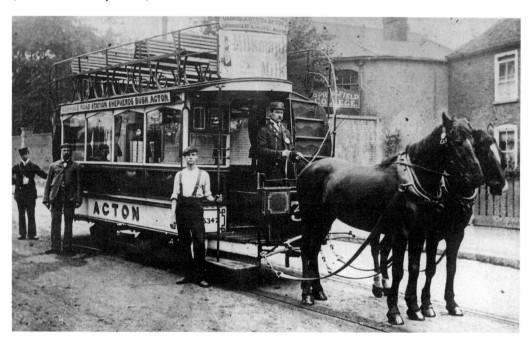

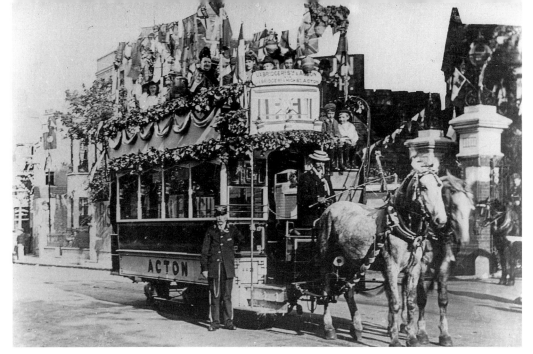

39.  An LUT horse tram, built by G.F.Milnes & Co Ltd, stands outside Acton Depot, gaily decorated in honour of Queen Victoria's Diamond Jubilee on 20th June 1897. Everybody, everywhere was in festive mood that day.   (Dave Jones Coll.)

Acton Depot is shown on the 1914 edition, as is the LGOC's Bus depot.

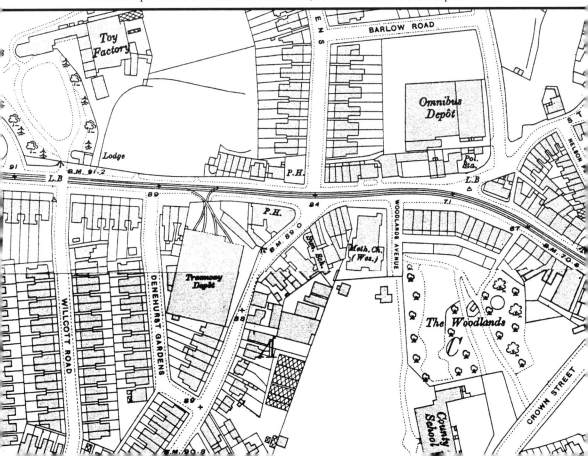

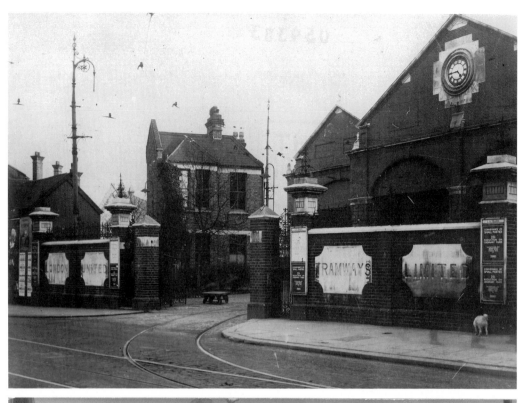

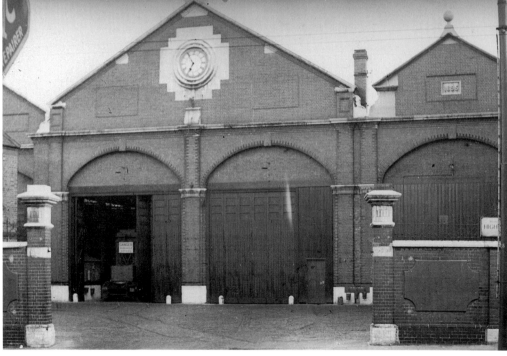

40. We view the entrance and left hand side of Acton Depot in about 1927. The building is situated on the south side of Uxbridge Road, between Gunnersbury Lane and Denehurst Gardens. The four concrete panels in the red brick front wall, reading LONDON UNITED TRAMWAYS LIMITED, still exist. Posters outside proclaim CONVEYANCE OF SMALL PARTIES - 25% REDUCTION ON ORDINARY FARES.  (LUT)

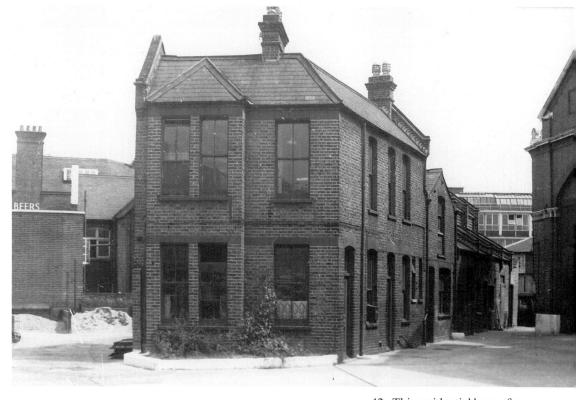

41. Acton Depot dates back to 1895 and was enlarged in 1900; it still survives and is pictured here on 11th May 1951. It ceased to house tramcars in 1936, but is still known as the "Tram Depot", and buses terminating here display "Acton Tram Depot" on their destination blinds. It housed trolleybuses for three months in 1936 after the 89 route to Hammersmith had been converted. Acton never supplied trolleybuses for the main Uxbridge route 607. From 12th September 1937 it ceased to house trolleybuses, or motor buses either, and for the next 53 years it was used exclusively for overhead tower wagons and as a store for electrical equipment. On 26th May 1990 it reopened as a bus garage; the building subsequently displayed the legend Ealing Buses Acton Tram Depot.
(John Gillham)

42. This residential house for the depot superintendent was built by the LUT in 1895. Situated in the forecourt of Acton Depot, it was later used as offices, and this photo was taken on 30th June 1962. It was demolished in 1990 to provide extra parking space for another eight buses outside the main building.
(John Gillham)

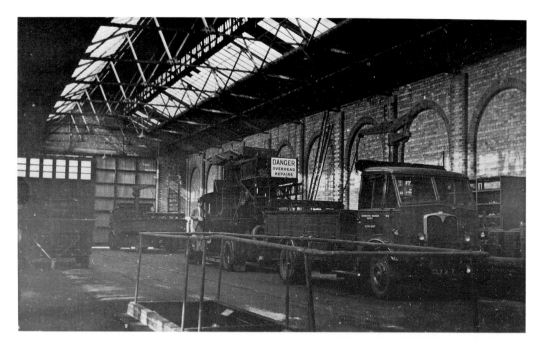

43. This is the interior of one of the four bays of Acton Depot. Looking towards the main doorway in 1938, we observe an AEC Mercury pole erecting lorry and an Associated Daimler tower wagon. (J.W.Stuchlik)

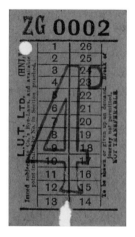

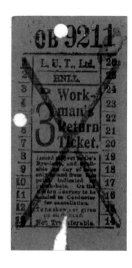

# EALING

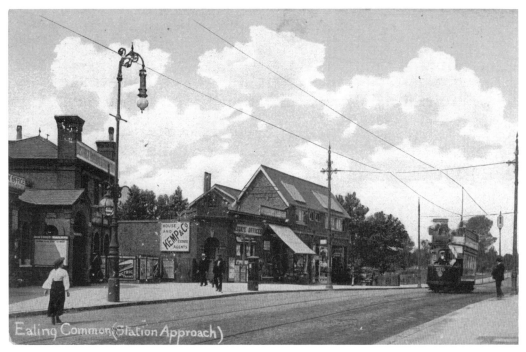

Ealing Common (Station Approach)

44. The boundary between the boroughs of Acton and Ealing was at Birch Grove. Car 210 is passing Ealing Common Station on the District Railway. The station opened in 1879 and was totally rebuilt in 1931.   (Commercial Postcard)

45. Surface water drainage in the old days was not as good as it is today. On the evening of 15th June 1903 there was a heavy storm, resulting in this flood on Ealing Common, with car 113 ploughing through it. Note the centre poles which Ealing Borough Council insisted upon for the whole route through its territory.   (Commercial Postcard)

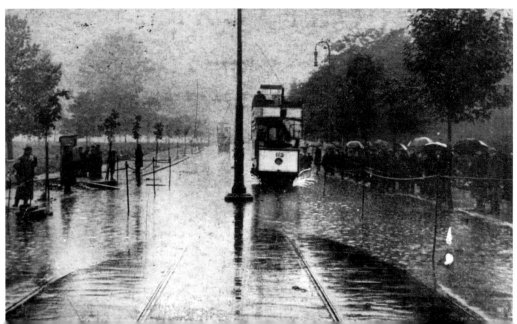

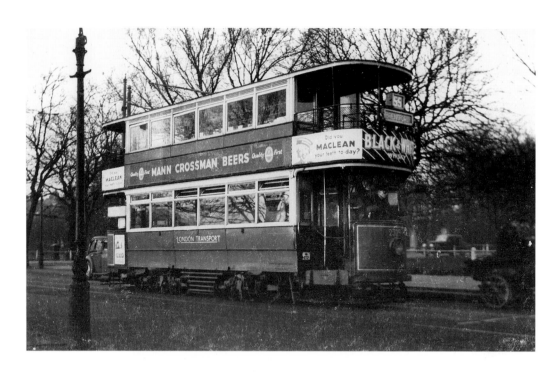

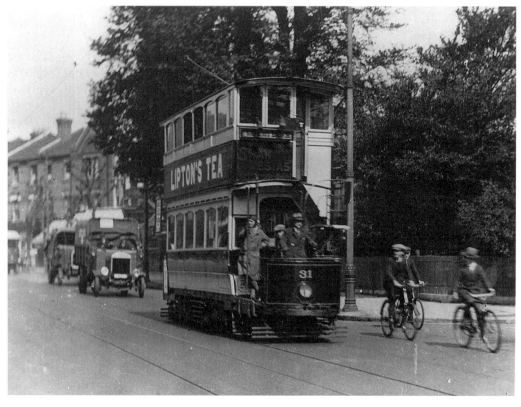

←⎯⎯⎯⎯⎯

46. T type car 313 after acquisition by the LPTB in 1933 was renumbered 2329, and it is seen here crossing Ealing Common. The destination blind shows 55 BRENTFORD, so it must be a Saturday. The basic 55 was Brentford to Hanwell, extended to Ealing in 1928, and later further extended across the Common to Acton on Saturdays only. This was confusing because the LGOC had its own bus route in the area, numbered 55, totally different, but also serving Hanwell, Ealing and Acton by other roads. (M.N.A.Walker)

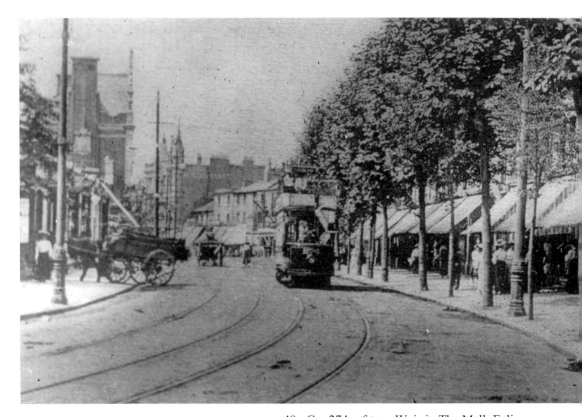

←⎯⎯⎯⎯⎯

47. Y type tram 31 travels eastwards from The Mall on to Ealing Common, opposite the end of Hamilton Road. The motorman is out of uniform, so he may be a "volunteer" drafted in during the General Strike of May 1926. A Thornycroft army lorry follows behind. The buildings in the distance still exist, but the trees have now been replaced by three blocks of flats. (A.D.Packer Coll.)

48. Car 274, of type W, is in The Mall, Ealing, with the end of Windsor Road in the distance. (Commercial Postcard)

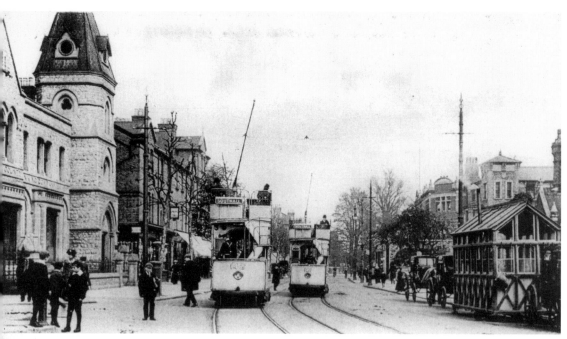

49. We look east along The Mall before 1908, with Station Approach off to the left. The imposing building on the left, opposite cars 142 and 121, is a bank and it still exists, as do most of the buildings visible here. (Commercial Postcard)

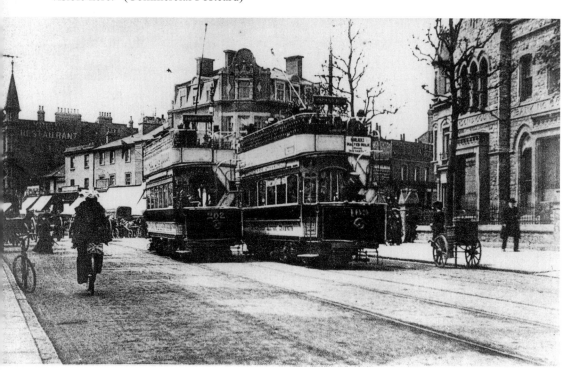

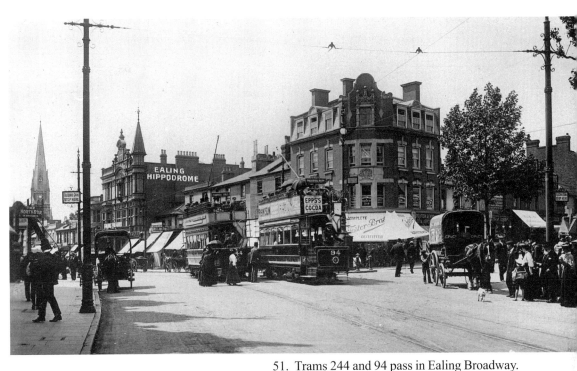

50. Looking west along The Mall from Windsor Road, we catch sight of cars 202 and 109. Both of these vehicles are now painted red. The Railway Station Approach is on the right beyond the bank; the road beyond here becomes The Broadway. (Commercial Postcard)

51. Trams 244 and 94 pass in Ealing Broadway. The Hippodrome was originally The Lyric, but was demolished a long time ago and replaced by new retail shops. Most of the other buildings are still substantially the same, and Foster Bros, to the right of car 94, occupied this corner for 50 or more years. Your author's parents bought his school uniforms there. The spire on the extreme left belongs to Christ Church. (Commercial Postcard)

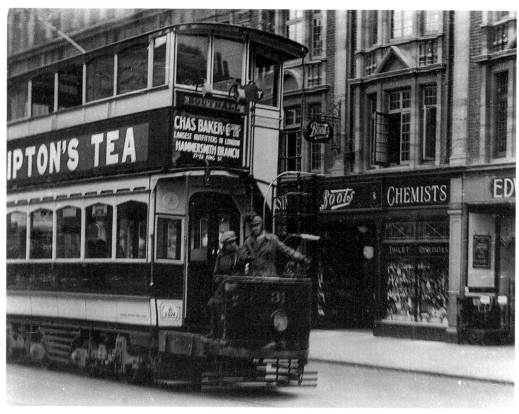

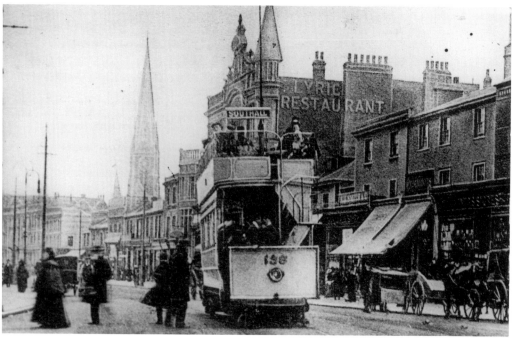

52. This is the point where The Mall becomes The Broadway, exactly opposite Station Approach, and we are looking south. Car 31, whose opposite end we saw in picture 47, is making a return journey to Southall, again with a driver out of uniform.   (A.D.Packer Coll.)

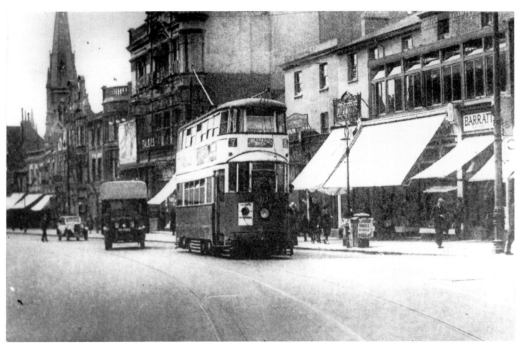

54. We move on another 28 or 30 years from the previous view, but we are at exactly the same spot. Note the modern tramcar, type UCC car 377, built in 1931.  (Commercial Postcard)

53.  Ealing Broadway looking west, with tram 138; Oxford Road is on the bottom left, and the spire of Christ Church is in the distance. All the properties on the right have now had their fronts altered. The Lyric has been replaced by W.H.Smith, and most of those beyond have been demolished and replaced by new buildings. (Commercial Postcard)

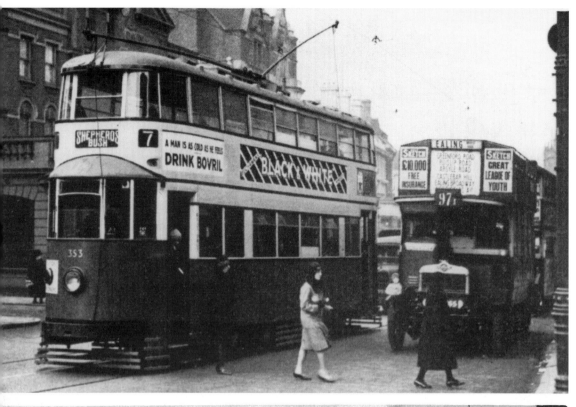

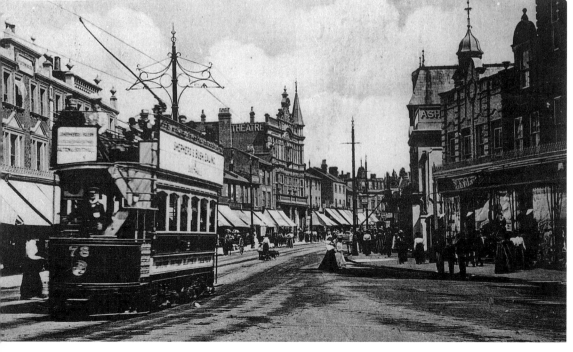

55. Ealing Broadway in 1931 and Feltham car 353 shows four passengers alighting from its front exit, while others board at the rear. A General K type bus is held up on its journey from Brentford Half Acre to Argyle Road in the extreme north of Ealing. (LUT)

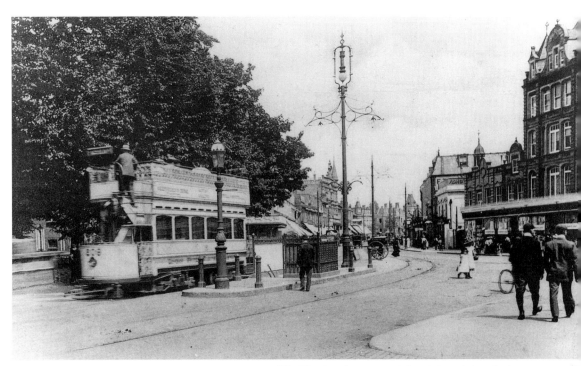

57. Plenty of ornamental metalwork to admire here as we observe car 208 in pristine condition. The grounds of Christ Church are on the left and in the centre of the picture is a very ornamental lamp atop an equally intricate traction pole. Note the public convenience on an island between the two tram tracks. This was an essential facility which was demolished and filled in sometime around 1980. (Dave Jones Coll.)

56. We find ourselves at the far end of Ealing Broadway and we look back eastwards to Z type tram 78. Note the ornamental traction standard which seems to be sprouting out of the top of the tram! (Commercial Postcard)

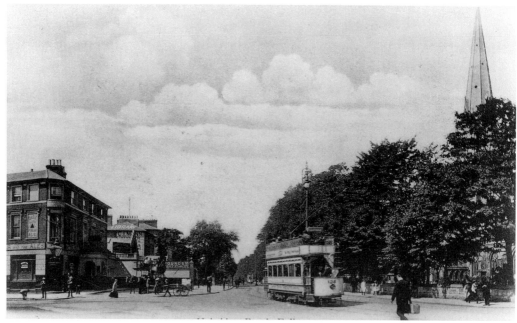

58. Looking west again, from the end of The Broadway in the very early days, we see car 128 and New Broadway in the centre, Christ Church on the right, and High Street on the left. The Railway Hotel on the left, with its granite setted forecourt, was a bus terminus for many years, but everything on the left was demolished in recent years and replaced by a parade of modern retail shops. (J.L.E.Perkins Coll.)

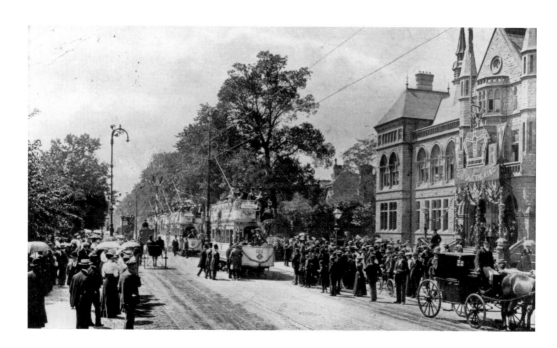

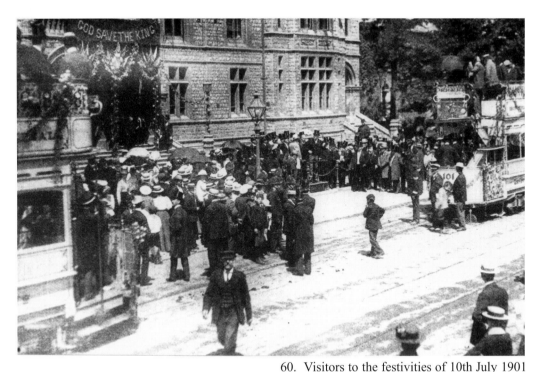

60. Visitors to the festivities of 10th July 1901 included ten peers, eight knights, six MPs, most of the members of eleven local borough or urban district councils, many managers and directors of tramways elsewhere, especially Bristol, railway officials, electrical experts, C.C.Cramp who had leased the horse tramway in 1876, and the editors or representatives of 64 newspapers and journals. Lord Rothschild, who lived locally in Gunnersbury Park, officially declared open all the tramways in West London and Middlesex - for the second time - he had already done the same at Shepherds Bush at twelve noon. A.J.Balfour, who became Prime Minister a year later, also made a speech. Nobody mentioned the fact that, during the three months of LUT electric operation, East Ham Corporation had *officially* opened its first electric line on 22nd June. (Commercial Postcard)

←——————

59. Ealing Urban District Council had arranged its Charter of Incorporation as a Borough (The first in Middlesex) to be celebrated on Wednesday, 10th July 1901. The LUT opened its tramway extension from Acton Hill to Southall Town Hall on the same day for one enormous combined celebration. Nine cars (101-109), of the brand new type X, were chosen to carry the 450 important guests in a grand procession. The nine trams ran empty from Hanwell Depot to Shepherds Bush, there they loaded all the guests, departed at twelve noon, took them out to Southall, and then back as far as Ealing. Here the VIPs alighted for a ceremony on the steps of the Town Hall, as seen in this picture, before being taken back to Shepherds Bush, and thence down Goldhawk Road to Chiswick Tram Depot. Here they inspected the power station and partook of a sumptuous banquet at 2pm. (Commercial Postcard)

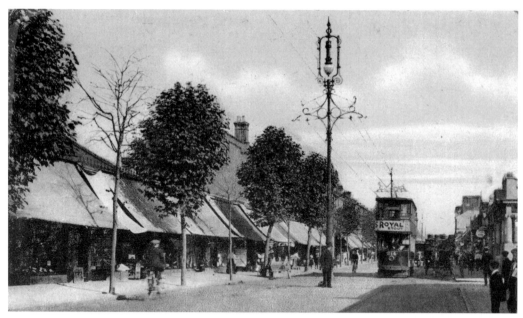

61. In Uxbridge Road, West Ealing, looking east from Northfield Avenue, we see car 314 at the end of Chapel Road. Ealing Urban District Council had insisted that the whole of its section of route must have the traction poles in the centre of the road, instead of at the sides with span wires like everybody else. The LUT certainly produced some magnificent poles, half of them with a lamp on top as well, but with the growth of motor traffic they became an obstruction, and they were removed only a few years later. All the buildings on the right of this picture still exist, but the low ones on the left have been supplanted by new four storey shops.   (Commercial Postcard)

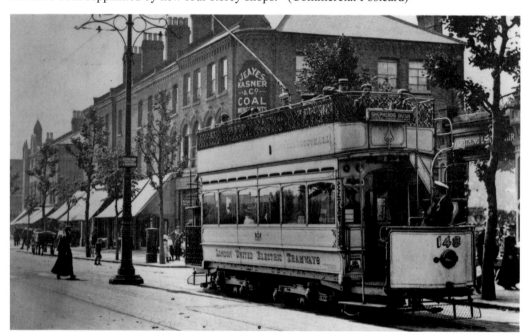

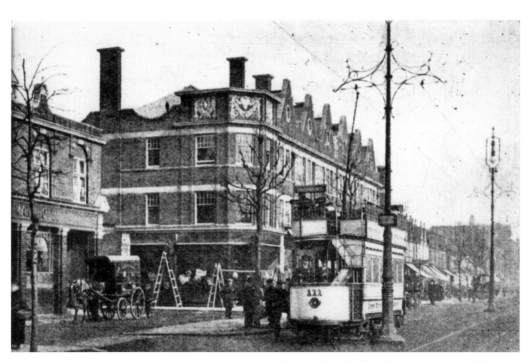

63. In West Ealing Broadway, car 111 stops outside the Green Man Hotel. This was demolished around 1990.
(Commercial Postcard)

←————————

62. We look west from the same spot as in the previous view. Northfield Avenue leads off to the left, and Drayton Green Road to the right. This point was always known as Kasner's Corner, because of the local coal merchant. The ELECTRIC CARS STOP HERE signs, by being mounted on the centre poles, served for both directions. All the buildings visible here still exist. (Middlesex County Times)

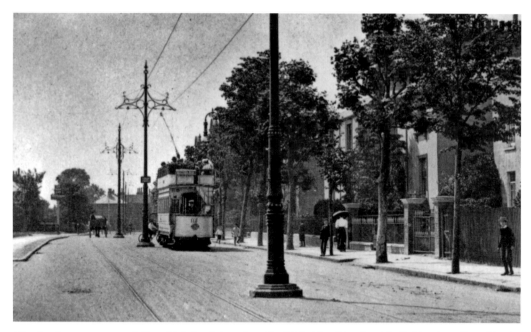

64. Again we espy car 111, which is pictured on the Uxbridge Road, with Coldershaw Road in the bottom left corner. The buildings in the distance are still there, but the pub on the left has gone. This view dates from before 1905 when the big houses on the right were replaced by shops. (Middlesex County Times)

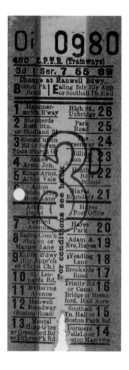 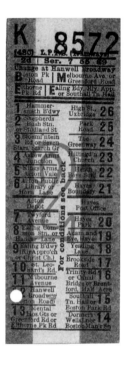

# HANWELL

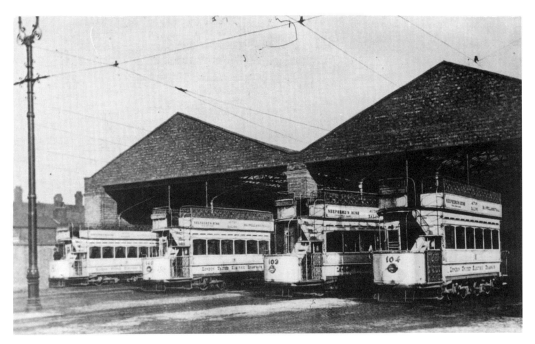

65.  The previous picture is within a few yards of the municipal boundary, at Grosvenor Road, between Ealing and Hanwell. Another third of a mile brings us to Hanwell Tram Depot, on the south side of Hanwell Broadway. This facility was a much larger one than Acton and lay parallel to the main road, but mostly hidden by retail shops. Access was by way of a fairly narrow entrance followed by a right angle corner. X type cars 104, 103, 146 and another are depicted in front of the original depot. In view of the fact that the LUT made such attractive ornamental structures of its depots at Acton, Chiswick, Hounslow and Fulwell, it is surprising that Hanwell possessed only the plainest brickwork. This picture is looking east.   (John Gillham Coll.)

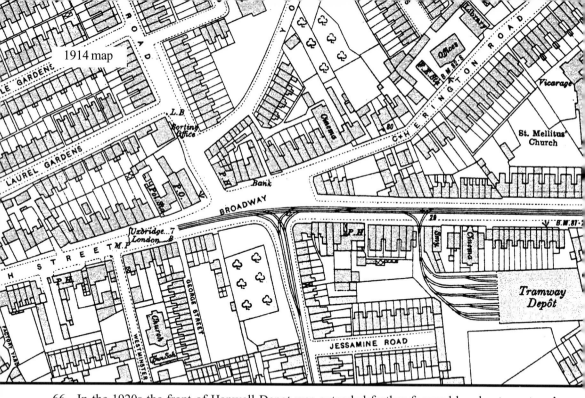

1914 map

66. In the 1920s the front of Hanwell Depot was extended further forward by about one tram's length, on each of ten tracks. Two open air tracks were added on the right hand side, and the extension was finished in corrugated iron. The houses visible in the distance were in Montague Avenue, and still exist. This picture was taken on 29th June 1935, but soon afterwards the houses were hidden when the depot building was further enlarged to cover the whole of the open ground in this picture. Trolleybuses operated here from 1936. This picture also shows the LUT Engineering and PW car 005, and car 148, an X type car which escaped being scrapped when most of the other members of the class were disposed of in 1922. Car 148 was repainted dark grey and converted into a sweeper and vacuum cleaning car. Its destination blind reads DEPOT ONLY.   (D.W.K.Jones)

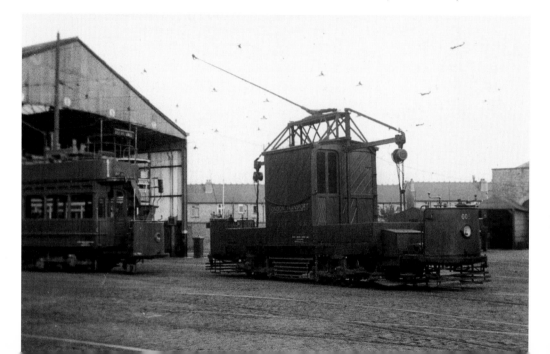

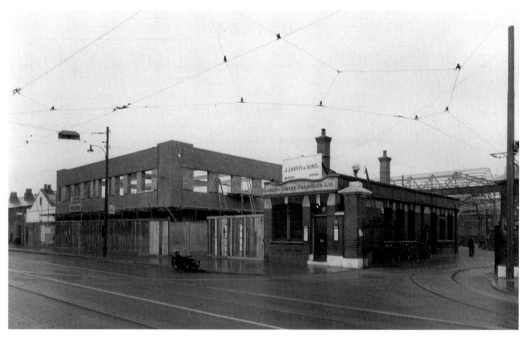

67. Hanwell Depot is depicted in the throes of conversion to trolleybuses in October 1936. The former LUT office block of 1901 is in the centre; it was a pity that this attractive building was demolished. On the left a much larger new building is being erected with offices downstairs and a staff canteen upstairs. In the background the steel framework of the depot extension for the future trolleybuses can be seen.   (LPTB)

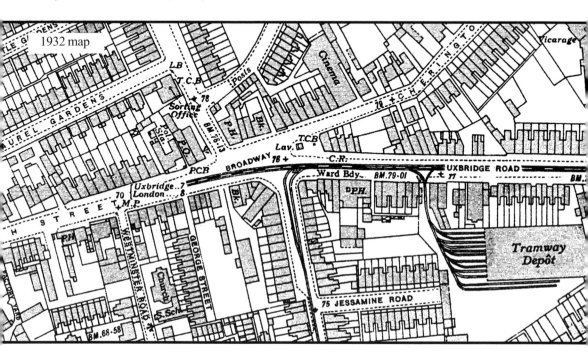

1932 map

68.   The interior of the depot shows the roof trusses above the lines of condemned trolleybuses. This depot held trams for 36 years, trolleybuses for 24 years and diesel buses for 33 years, before closure in April 1993. The whole structure, including the new office block, was demolished in the spring of 1996.
(John Gillham)

69. Hanwell Broadway is on the right, just a few yards west of the depot, with two trams passing. Cherington Road goes off to the left, and Boston Road to the right. The building in the background still survives, but J.C.Vaux has become of a micro centre of high technology.
(Commercial Postcard)

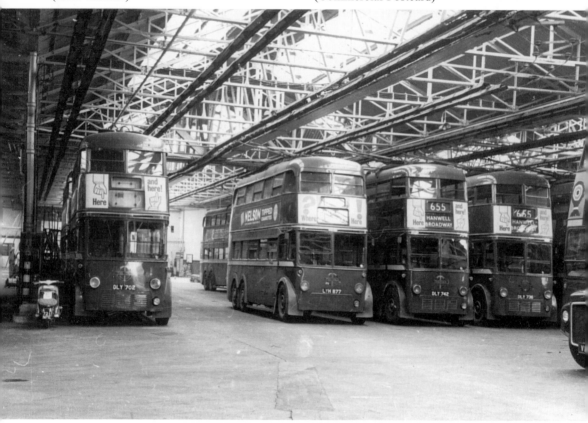

70. For most of its life the Boston Road service was worked as a self contained local shuttle between Hanwell and Brentford. No regular service ever used the junction curve at Brentford, and that at Hanwell was only employed after 1928 and for depot access. From 2nd September 1925 to 8th November 1928 the service was worked by four, one man operated, front entrance single deckers. To aid the single operator of each car, trolley reversers were installed at both termini. Many new housing estates were built in or near Boston Road in the 1920s and passenger traffic increased so much that route 55 reverted to double deckers on 9th November 1928. Some years later even Felthams took a turn on Sundays. This picture shows car 342 in the depot forecourt in 1925.  (LUT)

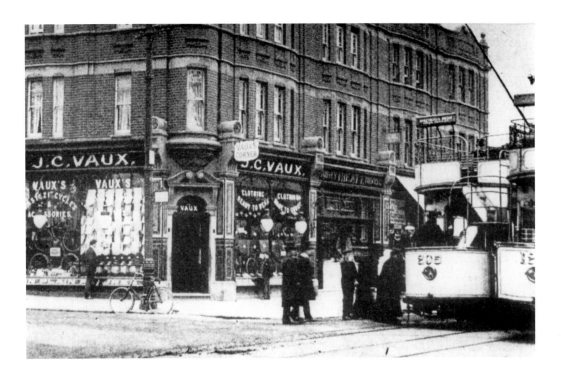

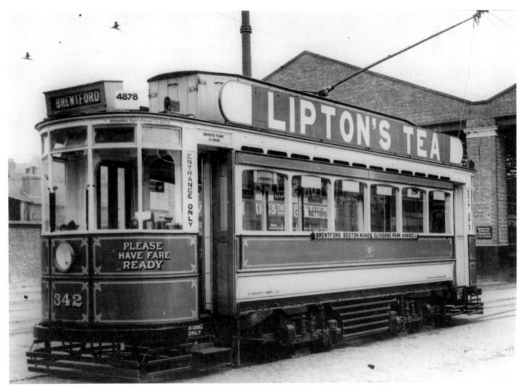

71. Cars 342-344 were designated type S2, and were cut down type W cars. Here we observe the front entrance of car 344. It had air operated doors on both sides. Behind the driver and to his left there was a fare box at waist height, worked by a foot pedal, and a second pedal operated a ticket punch. The driver had a rotating seat, a glass windscreen, a windscreen wiper, and an air brake control with "deadman" attachment. In those days, contrasting with the almost universal "one person operated" practice of modern times, it was extremely rare to run a tram (or a bus) without a conductor. (LUT)

→ 72. The rear exit of car 344 shows the door, which opened automatically when a passenger stood on a treadle plate inside the car. Internally this tram seated 32 on two full length longitudinal benches. (LUT)

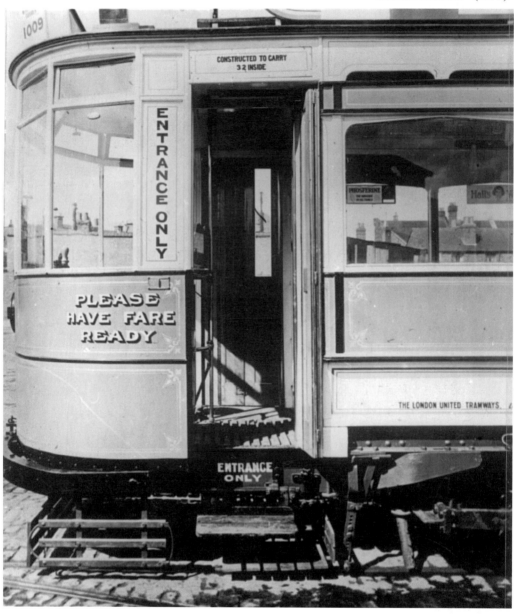

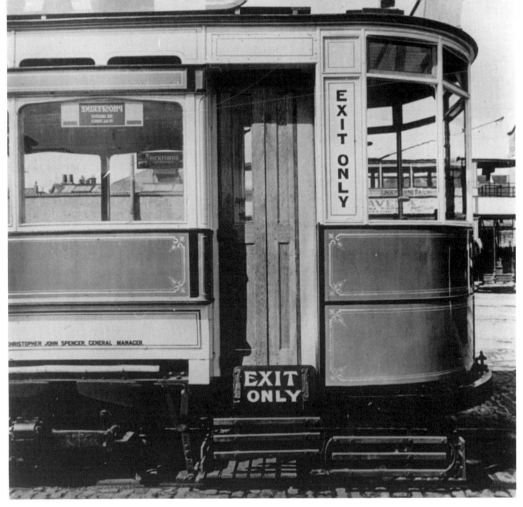

73. We encounter car 344 again, this time at the terminus at the Hanwell end of Boston Road; we are looking south. These cars had no provision for displaying their route number, and their destination blinds were never normally altered.   (George Gundry)

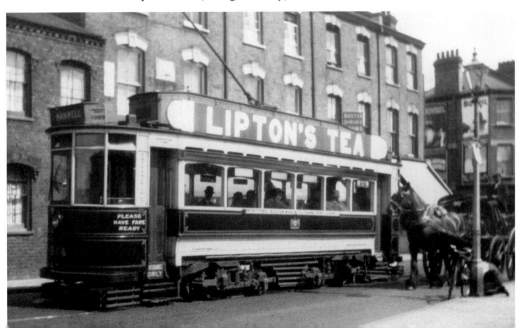

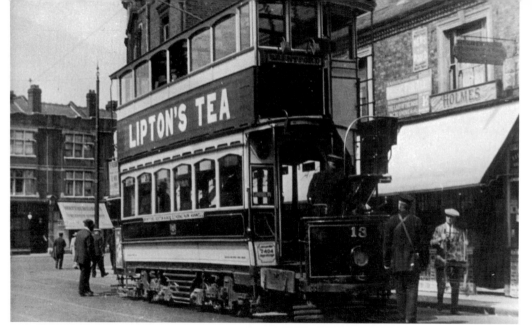

74. Three Y type double deckers were kept at Hanwell for augmenting the single deckers at rush hours. All the other 97 members of types Y and Z normally worked in the Kingston area. This photo shows a Y at Boston Road terminus, looking north, with Uxbridge Road in the distance. All the buildings here still exist. (Frank Merton Atkins)

75. We are in Boston Road, looking north, at the junction where the normal service went to the right to the terminus. To the left is Lower Boston Road where tracks were laid in 1906. A long through service ran at first from Hammersmith via Brentford and Lower Boston Road to Uxbridge. This was soon cut back to Southall and ceased by 1910. After this date the rails in Lower Boston Road fell into disuse and they were removed in 1930. The date of this picture is around 1932-33. (D.W.K.Jones)

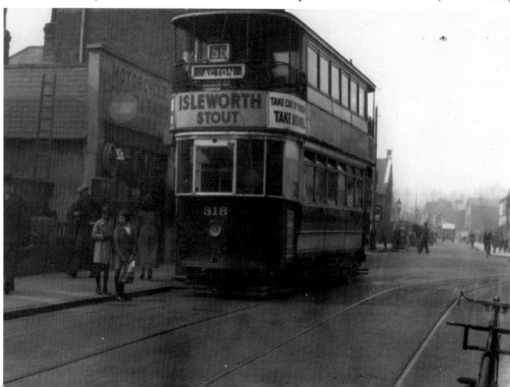

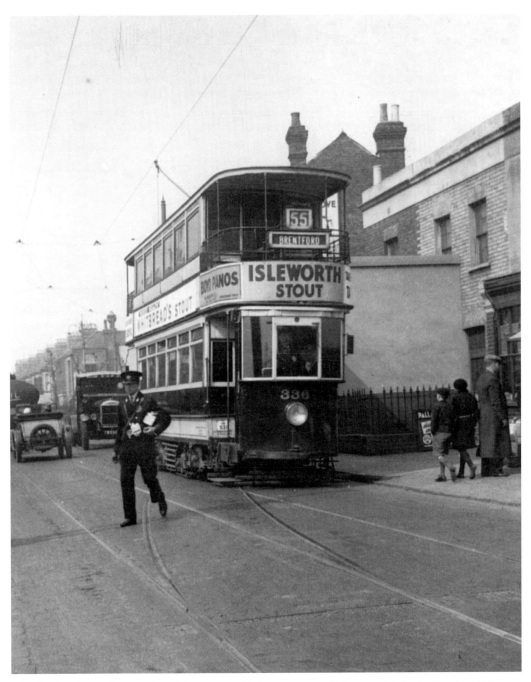

76. Further down Boston Road there was a facing crossover between Oaklands Road and Humes Avenue. It is assumed that this is the same location. We can speculate as to the reason why the conductor of car 336 was taking his ticket box with him as he crossed the road. Perhaps he was about to buy a newspaper or some cigarettes at the shops featured in the next picture. The date is 1932-33. (G.N.Southerden)

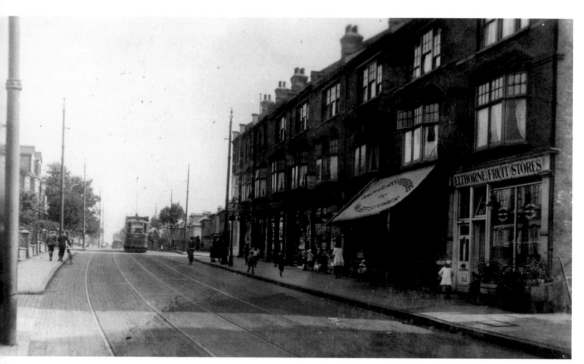

77. Boston Road, looking south between Oaklands Road and Cumberland Road, with car 341 in the distance. We assume that the facing crossover is just behind the cameraman. (R.J.Harley Coll.)

78. Car 341 (fully described in companion volume *Kingston and Wimbledon Tramways*) is seen in Boston Road opposite Clitherow Avenue and Chepstow Road, sometime between 1925 and 1928. All the houses, also the brick pillar on the extreme right, are still the same in 1998. The Church Hall in the picture has since been replaced by a new brick built structure, and a splendid new church, St.Thomas's, was built in 1933 between the Hall and the first house. (A.D.Packer Coll.)

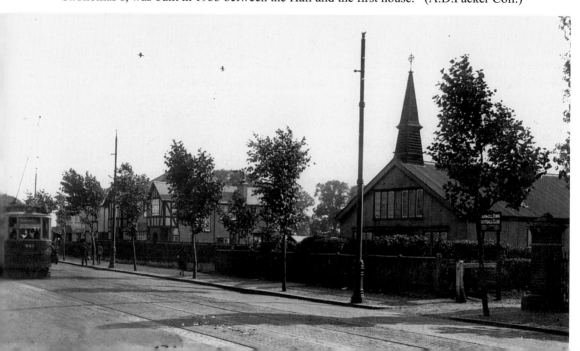

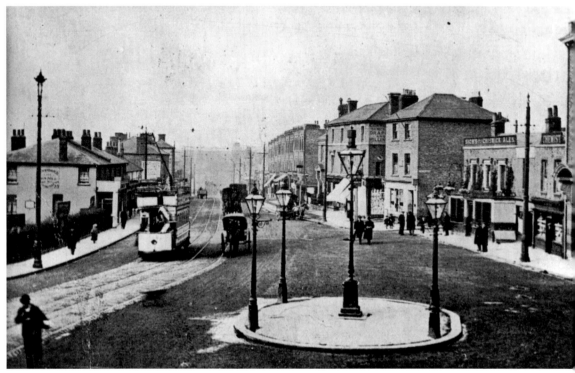

79. We return to Uxbridge Road and look west from the Vaux shop in photo 69 down the hill towards the River Brent. The island with five lamps was replaced in the 1930s by a clock tower and public convenience. Station Road, leading to the GWR Hanwell Station, goes off just beyond the Duke of York on the right. (Middlesex County Times)

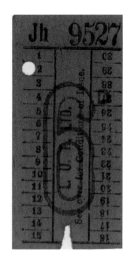

# SOUTHALL

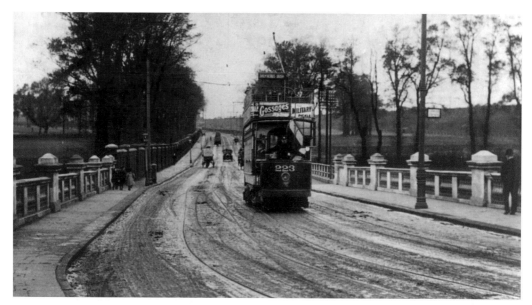

80. Car 223 proceeds on its journey to Shepherds Bush. Brent Bridge over the River Brent is the boundary between Hanwell and Southall. Wharncliffe Viaduct on the GWR is visible on the right, and the fields between it and the main road were covered in 1936 by a new housing estate. The land on the left belongs to Hanwell Mental Asylum, and around 1980 a huge new hospital was built here. (John Gillham Coll.)

81. A prominent feature on our trunk tram route is the Iron Bridge, where we pass under the four track main line of the Great Western Railway. When the railway was opened in 1838, there was indeed an iron bridge here, but it was soon replaced by one in steel, however, the old name is still used. We are looking west, with an open top tram in the far distance. Windmill Lane is on the left, with Greenford Road on the right beyond the bridge. (Commercial Postcard)

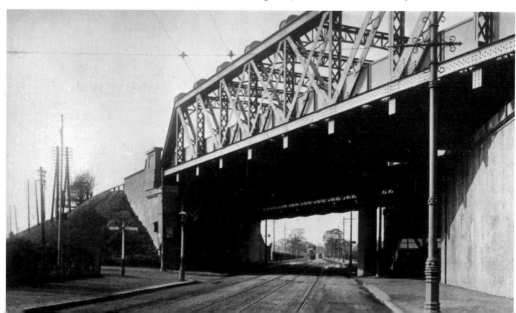

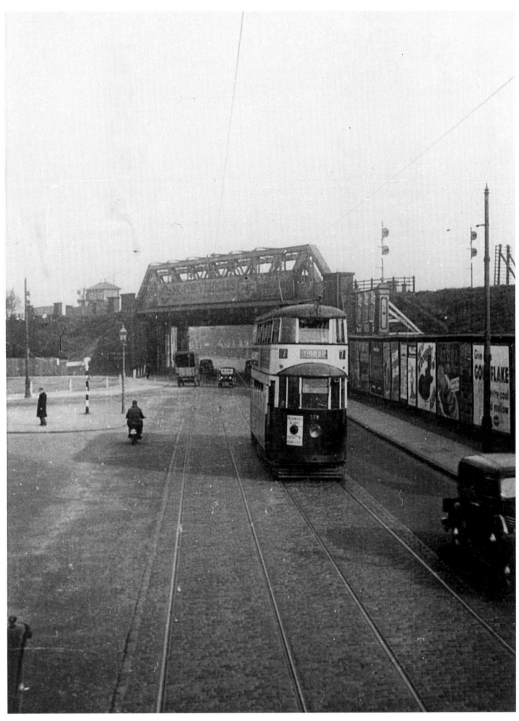

82. Beyond the Iron Bridge, we turn round and look back eastwards in about 1931-33, and we catch sight of Feltham car 378 on its way to Uxbridge. (G.N.Southerden)

83. Still further west, we see the Iron Bridge in the distance, with Feltham 379 on its way to the short working terminus at Southall Canal Bridge. We are in the country now, with the West Middlesex Golf Course on the left and Lyndhurst Avenue on the right. Circa 1930 a duplicate road, parallel to the tramway, was laid from the Iron Bridge as far as Southall Park. This was for motor vehicles to have a smooth, fast surface, thus avoiding the tram tracks and the granite setts; the two roads could be used in both directions! After tramway abandonment and removal of the rails, the keep left rule of the road was applied to the new dual carriageway. (C.Carter)

84. As we enter Southall High Street and look back to the east, we see an X type tram returning to London. The wall and trees on the right are of the grounds of the old Market House, where the Odeon Cinema was later built. The two pubs, the George and Dragon on the left, and the White Hart alongside the tram, were both later rebuilt on the same sites. (Middlesex County Times)

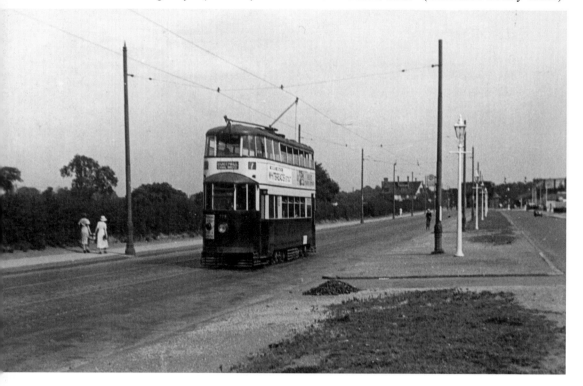

85. T type car 327 threads its way through Southall High Street, as we look to the east from the corner of South Road. Avenue Road is to the right of the horse and cart. The thoroughfare illustrated here was, and still is, a narrow, congested bottleneck. (Commercial Postcard)

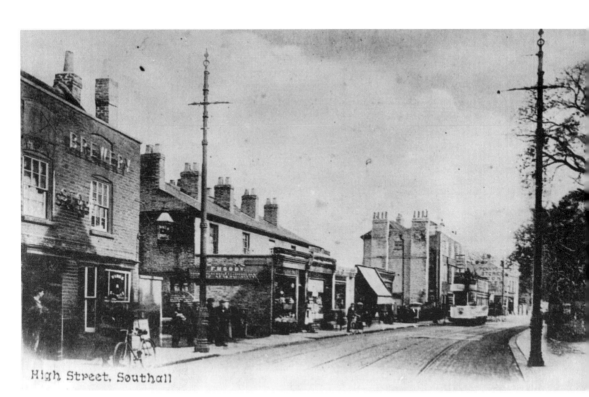

High Street, Southall

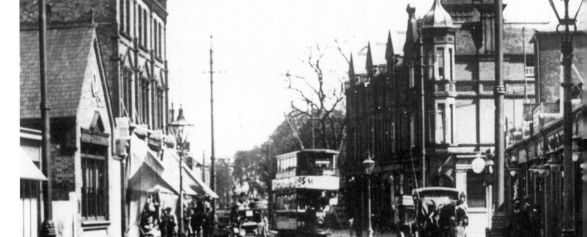

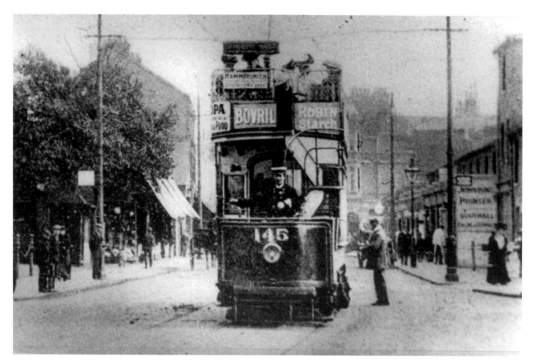

86. This tram in Southall High Street appears to be going to Shepherds Bush, according to the destination blind, although a route board seems to contradict this by suggesting that Hammersmith is the ultimate goal! South Road is off to the right and you can just see the railings of the Town Hall to the left. (Commercial Postcard)

87. Southall Town Hall, on the north side of the High Street by the corner of Lady Margaret Road, was where the tramway terminated on 10th July 1901. It was three years later before the rails were extended further. The Town Hall still exists, and is unchanged except that the glass canopy over the entrance steps has gone. Tram 336 is standing outside. (Commercial Postcard)

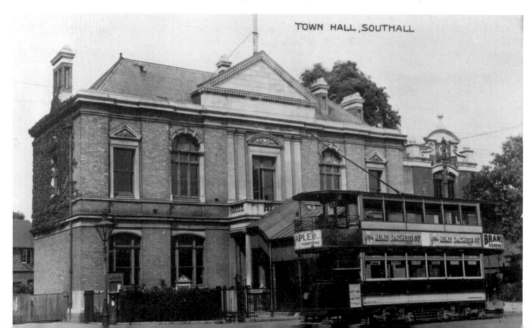

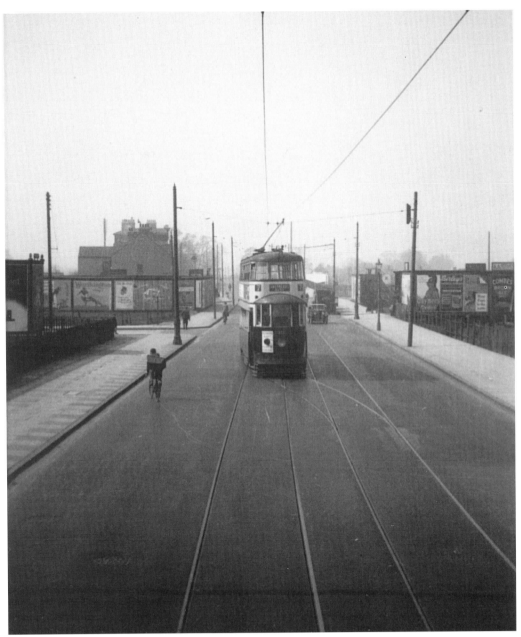

88. The whole of the 1904 extension was originally single track with 23 passing loops, and legally was a light railway and not a tramway. The section from Southall Town Hall to Yeading Brook on the Southall/Hayes boundary was later doubled, with two trailing crossovers. The service beyond Southall was always less frequent, and about half the trams turned back here - at various times at either the Town Hall, Townsend Road, Ranelagh Road or the Canal Bridge. The replacing 607 trolleybuses terminated at Delamere Road, mid way between the Canal Bridge and Yeading Brook. Here we look west to see Feltham car 352 reversing at Townsend Road. All the left side is now retail shops and the right side is residential flats and houses. (G.N.Southerden)

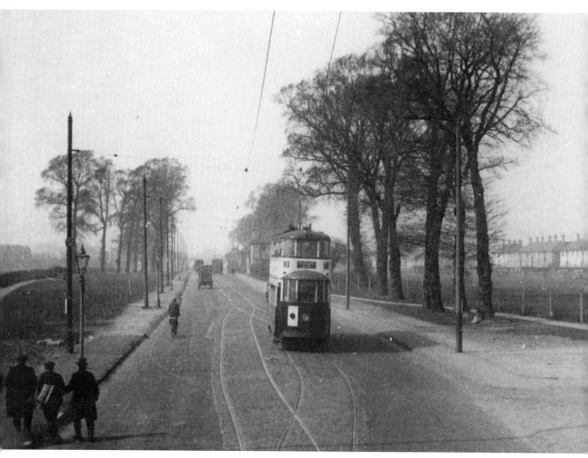

89.  At the far end of Southall we cross the Grand Junction Canal, and very soon afterwards the Yeading Brook is encountered. We shortly arrive at Brookside Road, where, looking west, we see a Feltham at a passing loop. It is strange that these fine, fast modern cars had to work on such an old fashioned and slow track layout. The rural peace of this view was shattered in the 1990s by the construction of a motorway style highway with a gigantic roundabout on the site of the former tram route.  (G.N.Southerden)

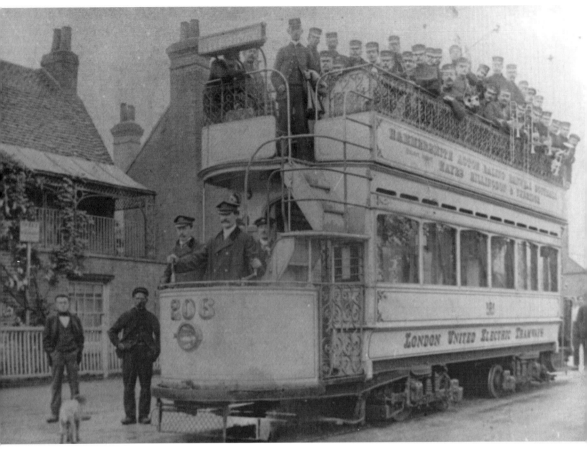

90. One mile from Brookside Road we reach the Adam and Eve public house, which in 1904 was an olde worlde country inn belonging to the small rural hamlet of Wood End. The pub itself is hidden by the tram in this picture, which was taken on 31st May 1904. The official inspection by Colonel Yorke of the Board of Trade took place with the help of car 202, of type W painted yellow. It travelled from Southall to Uxbridge, and behind it was white car 206 carrying the Uxbridge and Hillingdon Prize Brass Band, which played stirring music throughout the journey. Here we see them pausing for a moment outside the Adam and Eve. (Uxbridge Library)

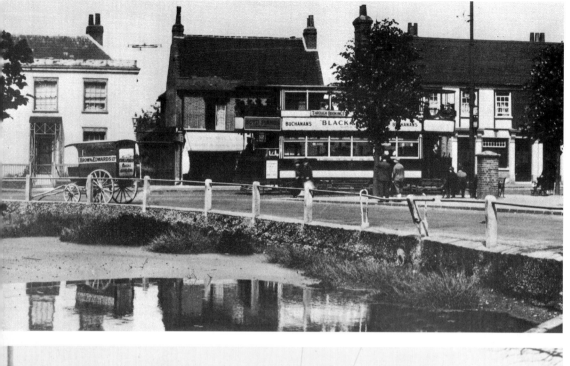

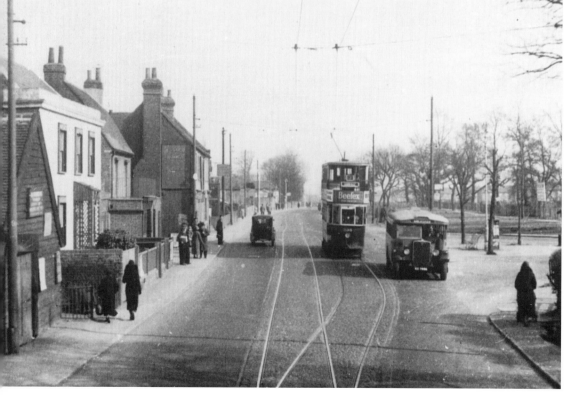

91. Much later, during the 1920s (because the route number 7 is displayed), we see a T type tram outside the Adam and Eve. Nothing from the past has yet changed in this picture, with the typical village duck pond on the other side of the main road. The Adam and Eve was rebuilt in 1937 as a modern pub and it now has some rather naughty, but very appropriate, pictorial sculptures in its stonework.   (Dave Jones Coll.)

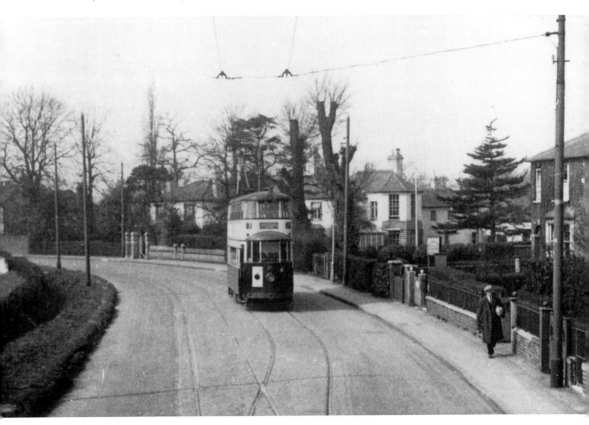

92. The Adam and Eve in this 1932 picture is the furthermost of the four large buildings. When rebuilt in 1937, it was relocated back from the road. Car 335 is on its way to Uxbridge. Church Road and the 98 bus route is off to the right. The AEC Regal coach is owned by the Amersham & District Motor Bus & Haulage Co Ltd, and it is seen on its regular run from Oxford Circus to Amersham via Shepherds Bush and Uxbridge. (G,N,Southerden)

93. Shortly beyond the Adam and Eve the old turnpike road made a detour to the north, which the LUT naturally had to follow in 1904. This was straightened out and by-passed in the late 1920s, so this part of the old tram route became a quiet backwater and was given the name of Park Road. Trams operated here right to the end, but the replacing trolleybuses used the by-pass. Here we are looking west at Feltham car 371 in Park Road, with Park Lane leading off to the right in the distance. Nowadays few would suspect that this was ever the main road to Oxford and a major tram route.   (A.D.Packer Coll.)

94. The town of Hayes is further to the south, but there was a small hamlet (now entirely built up) on the main road and tramway, known as Hayes End. It was centred around the White Hart Inn. In this picture, looking west, although the inn sign is on the left, the pub itself is on the right, alongside Z type car 57. Hayes End Road goes off to the right immediately beyond the White Hart. The White Hart itself still survives unaltered, but everything else has been swept away by a dual carriageway road.
(Alan Jackson Coll.)

95. A Feltham stands in front of the White Hart Inn. Note that even in LUT days some of the Felthams had two long advertising posters on each upper deck side. Some had one long poster in the middle flanked by two short ones. This advertising oddity was perpetuated through the Uxbridge Road period into the time when all Felthams were shedded at Streatham Depot. Nearly half a mile beyond the White Hart we cross the Hayes/Hillingdon boundary.
(J.W.Stuchlik)

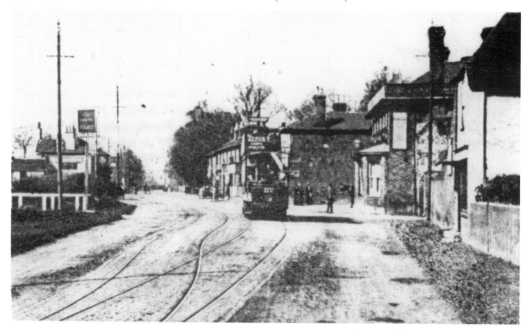

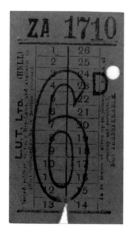

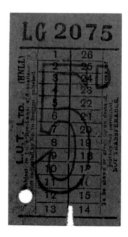

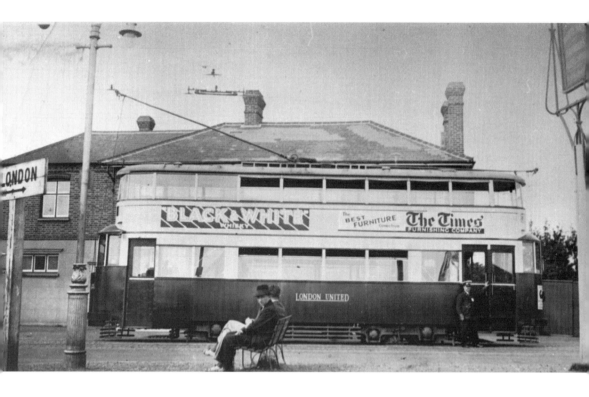

Hillingdon Depot on the 1916 survey.

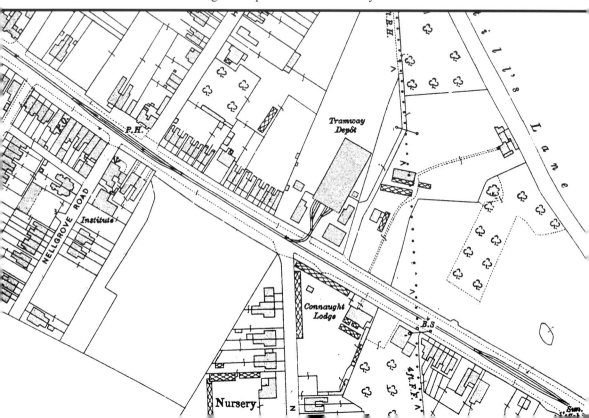

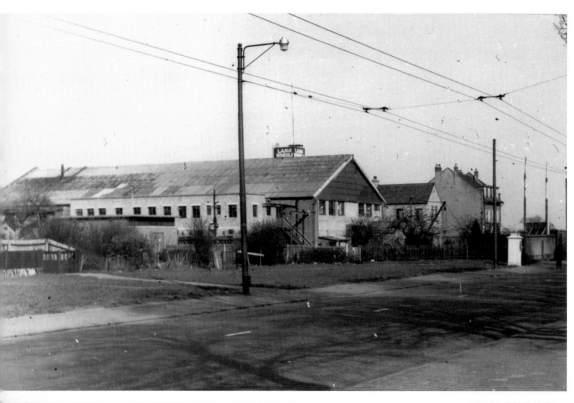

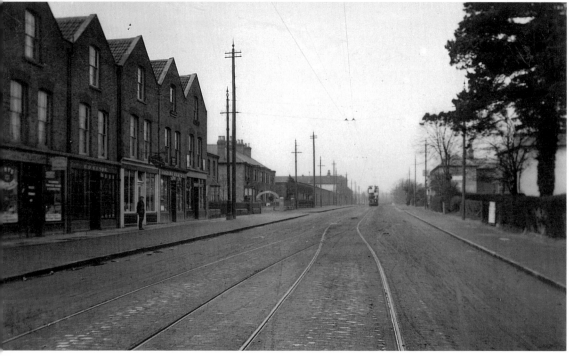

96. There was an LUT depot with five tracks at Hillingdon Heath, opposite the end of New Road. It was closed in 1922 and no photos of it have been located. The building was subsequently occupied by Lang Wheels Engineering, when this view was taken on 21st April 1951. The flat roofed building on the left was a trolleybus electrical sub-station. The site was cleared in late 1985 and a new block of flats was erected by January/February 1987.   (John Gillham)

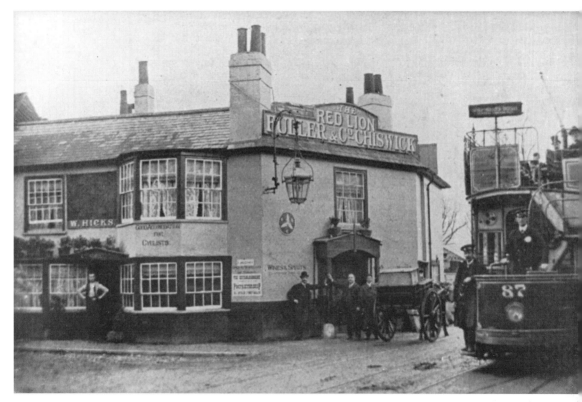

←————————

97.  Just beyond the depot, immediately west of Nellgrove Road, we see this passing loop with a tram in the distance. Everything on the right was demolished in the 1960s to make way for a dual carriageway. On the left everything in the distance has gone, but the nearer block of houses is still there. (A.D.Packer Coll.)

98.  The Red Lion in the centre of Hillingdon Village, opposite the Parish Church, still exists. The road is still narrow and twisty through the village. Royal Lane goes off to the left alongside the Red Lion. Immediately beyond, the old road and tramway down Hillingdon Hill was narrow, but a duplicate road was subsequently constructed on the right hand side as far as Stratford Bridge over the River Pinn, with a lovely avenue of trees between old and new highways.
(Uxbridge Library)

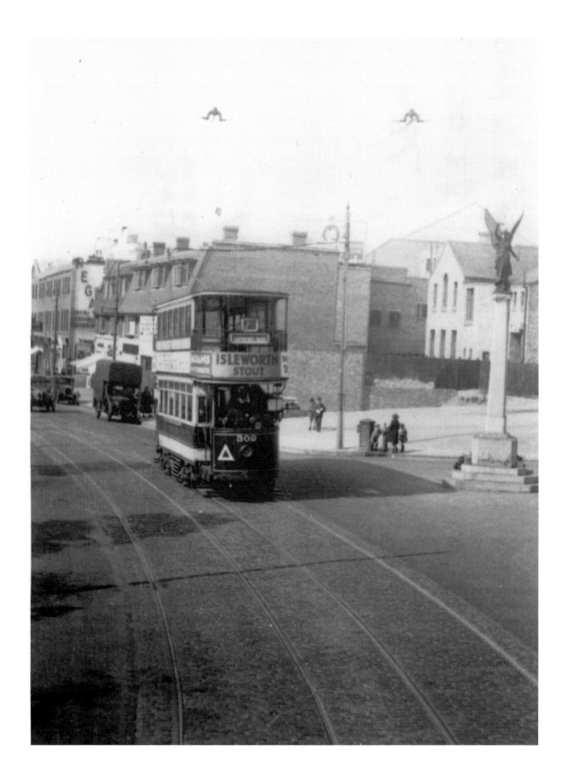

# UXBRIDGE

←————

99. Beyond the crossing of the River Pinn, the tramway curved around a large and important RAF depot. And thus we come to the south-east end of Uxbridge High Street, where we see car 309 passing the 1914-18 War Memorial. All the buildings visible still exist, but the War Memorial has gone, and there is now a huge traffic roundabout with a network of pedestrian subways. From here onwards, most of the High Street has been closed to all traffic, including buses. Most of the town centre, including the GWR station, to the left of this picture was demolished in 1965-70 for a new by-pass road. As a result, route 207 buses (successors to tram route 7 and trolleybus route 607) now have to make a mile diversion to reach their terminus outside the Metropolitan Railway Station - the trams were a lot more direct!   (A.D.Packer Coll.)

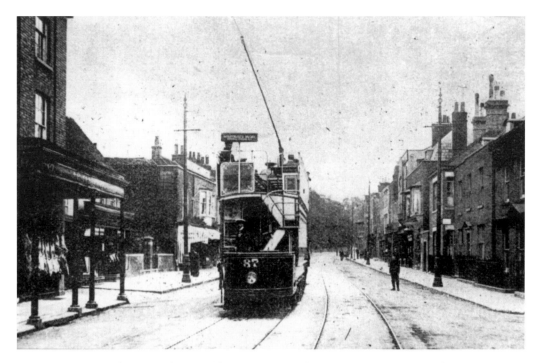

100. Tram 87, which we saw last at Hillingdon, is now in the south-eastern end of Uxbridge High Street. St.Andrew's Church is in the distance.   (John Gillham Coll.)

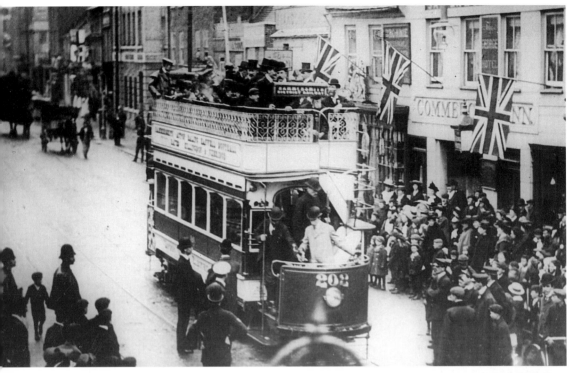

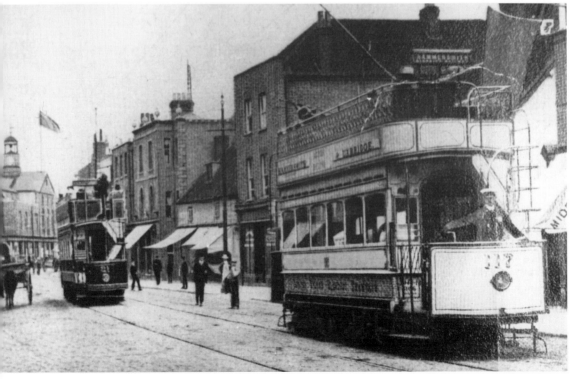

101. This view is dated 31st May 1904 and shows car 202 in Uxbridge High Street. This was certainly the date of the Board of Trade Inspection, which is known to have used car 202, but there seem to be too many passengers on board for that purpose. Probably the formal opening ceremony took place later the same day and using the same car, when a large party of VIPs was entertained to a grand banquet at the Chequers Hotel. But, despite the flags and crowds of spectators, the hotel on the right of the picture appears to be The George Hotel, Commercial Inn. It is recorded elsewhere that car 202 on 31st May was in yellow livery, but does the tram shown here look too dark? Incidentally, it shows HAMMERSMITH DISTRICT RAILWAY on its destination blind.  (Uxbridge Library)

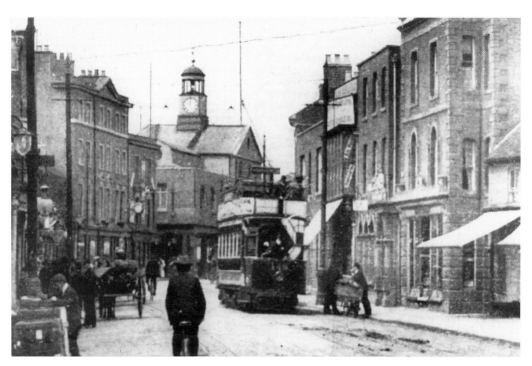

102. We look west to see car 21 passing car 117 in Uxbridge High Street. The tower in the distance on the left is the Market House. George Street is on the right, hidden by the tram.  (John Gillham Coll.)

103.  As we approach the Market House we pass tram 143. The buildings on the right have since been demolished, but the others are still there. Windsor Street on the left was once the main road to Windsor.  (Uxbridge Library)

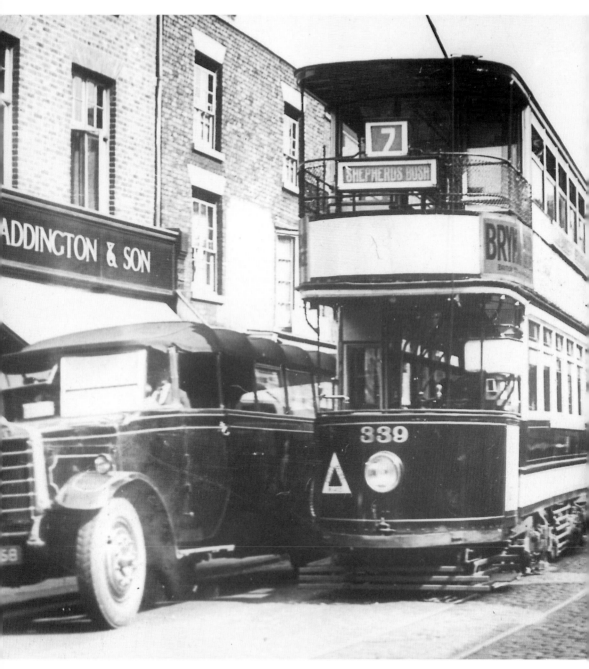

104. Traffic seems to be congested as a Daimler charabanc and a Leyland Lorry prove hazardous for two T type trams trying to squeeze past. We are looking east, with George Street on the left beyond car 339. The buildings visible here still exist, but Waddington & Son is now a charity shop. (Commercial Postcard)

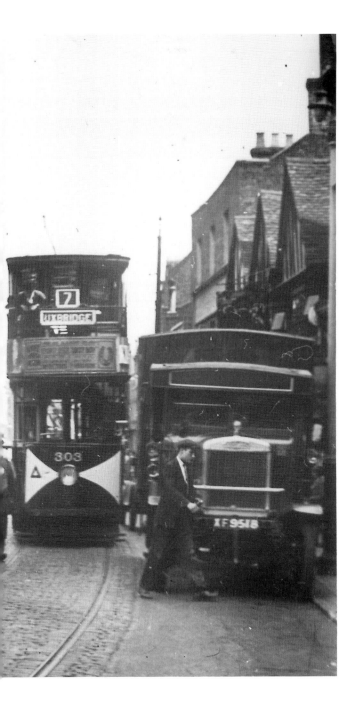

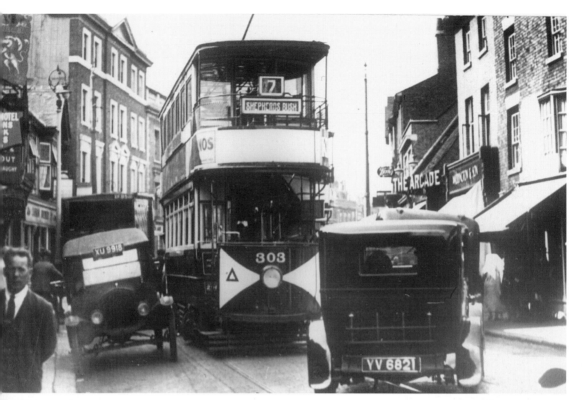

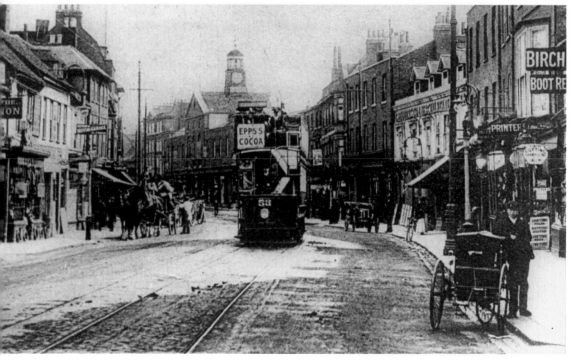

105. Car 303 in the previous picture has been to the end of the line and is now returning, but together with the ubiqitous Model T Ford van, it tempts two private saloon cars to explore the wrong side of the road. We again see Waddington, now on the right. The Kings Arms and the Three Tuns on the left still exist, but The Arcade now has a new front, and the building beyond it has gone. This picture is recorded as 31st October 1931, so we may assume that this date also applies to picture 104. (Commercial Postcard)

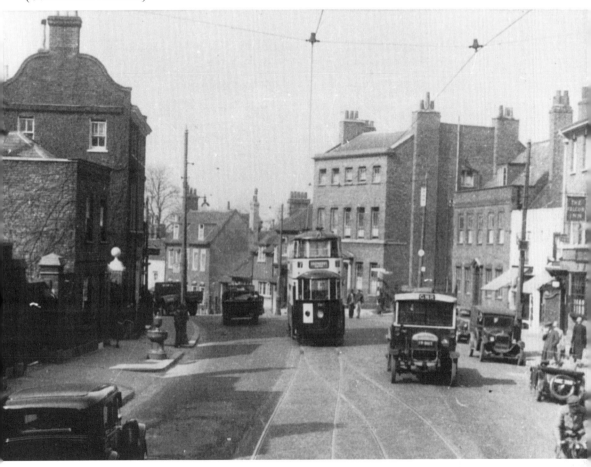

106. We have passed the Market House and now look back at it, as tram 53 approaches its terminus. All the buildings on the right this side of Market House, and all those on the left, were swept away in the mass destruction of 1960-80. There are many glass monstrosities here now, but the street is closed to all traffic, so drivers cannot see them! (Uxbridge Library)

107. At last we reach the terminus, and a Feltham is standing at the very end of the track, at the top of the short hill which leads down to Fray's River, the Grand Junction Canal and the River Colne, which marked the county boundary between Middlesex and Buckinghamshire. The road to Harefield is to the right of the tram, and we can just see an old style signpost. A GWR Thornycroft van is coming towards us. The buildings to the right of the van still exist, but the big one in the middle and all those down the hill have gone. (G.N.Southerden)

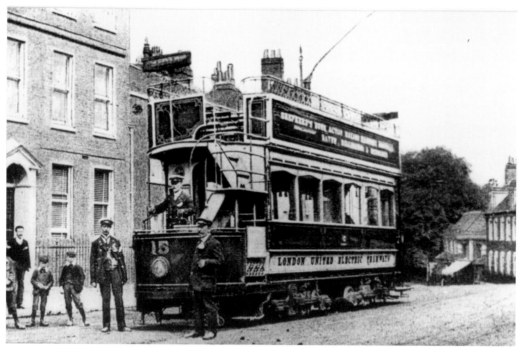

108. On 8th October 1908 a tram pauses at the terminus for a few minutes, before returning to Shepherds Bush, which will take 76 minutes. The driver, conductor, another driver, three children and a passer-by all pose to have their photograph taken. After a few years the description of the route on the top deck sides was replaced by commercial advertising posters. (Commercial Postcard)

109. In April 1933, car 356 stands at the same spot prior to making the same journey which now lasts only 67 minutes. The Fassnidge Memorial Hall on the left, with its porch, is still intact in 1998, but the building beyond it (hidden by the tram) has been demolished for a connecting road to the new by-pass. (M.J.O'Connor)

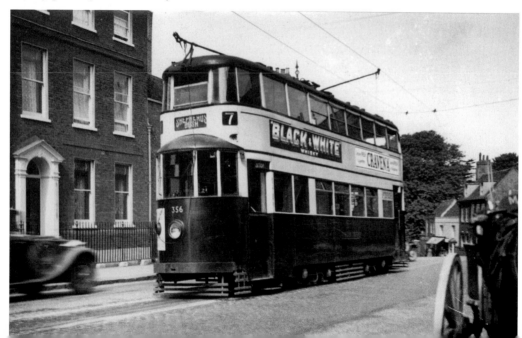

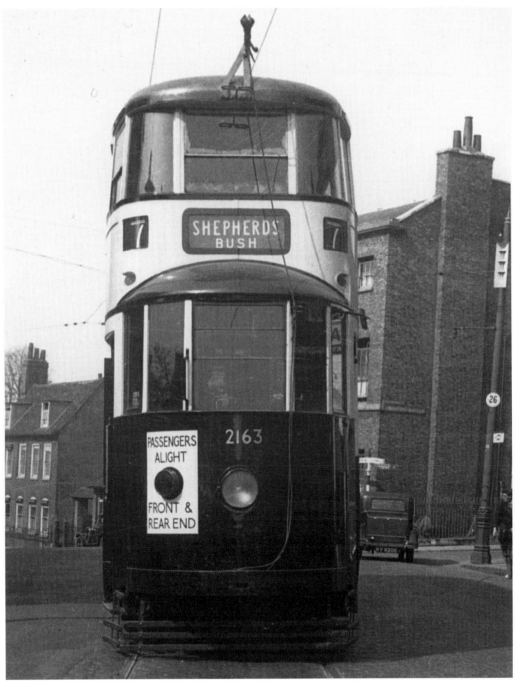

110. London Transport has now taken over, and car 2163, formerly LUT car 394, stands at the end of the track on 31st March 1934. Harefield Road is on the right. The High Street continued down the hill, and so did the trolleybuses, which went just a little bit further than the trams, to a specially built turning circle on private ground, all trace of which has now vanished. The 26 on the pole at the right is the fare stage number.   (G.N.Southerden)

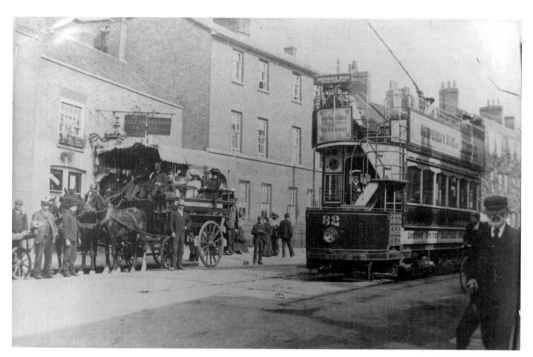

111. Immediately on the opening of the Uxbridge tramway, a Mr.Dunsby of the Plough Inn at Denham, inaugurated a service of horse wagonettes from the tram terminus to Denham Village. We presume this is his vehicle loading at the Falcon Inn. Car 82 displays SHEPHERDS BUSH & UXBRIDGE along the top deck sides, but other trams included references to Acton, Ealing, Hanwell, Southall, Hayes and Hillingdon on the displays. But in fact car 82 is out of bounds, because on the end panel it states SHEPHERDS BUSH CENTRAL LONDON RAILWAY & KEW BRIDGE, so we presume that underneath the detachable UXBRIDGE on the side panel, it says KEW BRIDGE. This may mean that Hanwell Depot has borrowed a tram from Chiswick Depot.   (Uxbridge Library)

112. We go a little way down the hill and look back to see car 205 loading.   (Commercial Postcard)

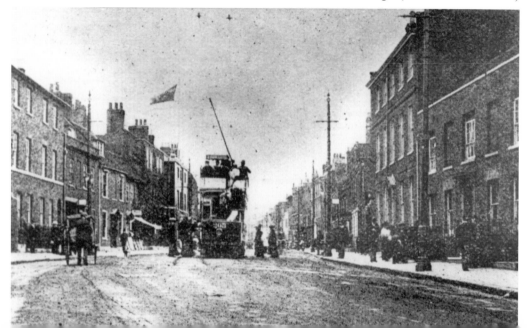

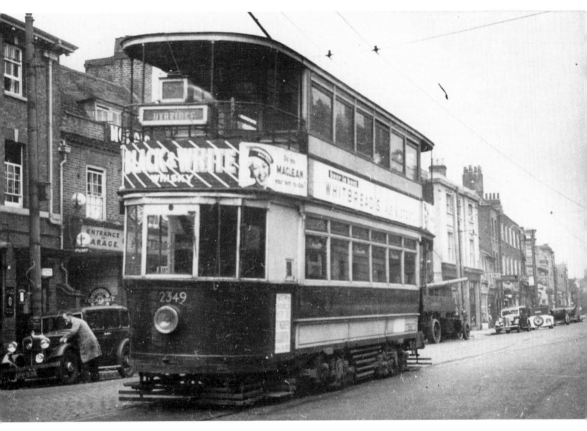

113. We can just see The Market House in the far distance past car 2349 (LUT car 333). Immediately beyond the tram we see the rear of a Foden steam pole-erecting wagon which is carrying new traction standards needed for the trolleybuses. Thus we finish our tram journey along the Uxbridge Road. (G.Freeze)

# ROLLING STOCK

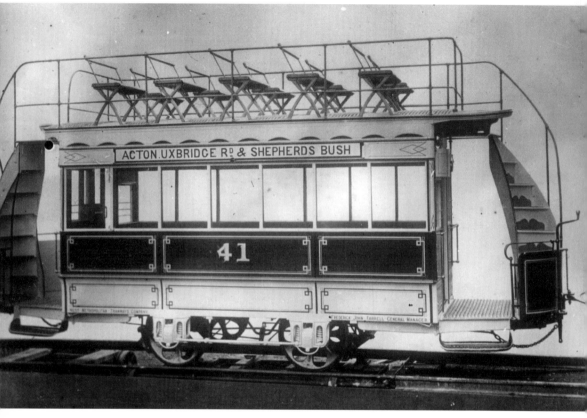

114. In the early days the SE&SB company had four cars, probably double decked. For its four routes the West Metropolitan bought a variety of single and double deck types, including toastracks, from at least three manufacturers. In 1886 for the Acton route they bought some garden seat cars from Falcon, as shown here. When the LUT took over in 1894, they bought some trams from Milnes, as shown in pictures 38 and 39, and later they built some themselves at Chiswick Depot. By the time of electrification in 1901 the total LUT horse tram fleet had risen to about 59 cars.  (Falcon Engine & Car Works)

## TYPE S2
Cars  342-344

Please refer to pictures 70, 71, 72 and 73 for illustrations of Type S2 cars

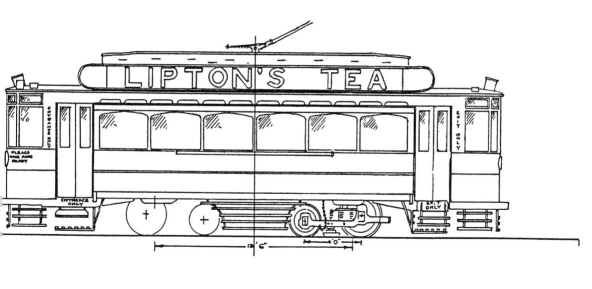

**LIPTON'S TEA**

PLEASE HAVE FARE READY

ENTRANCE ONLY

EXIT ONLY

13'6"     4'0"

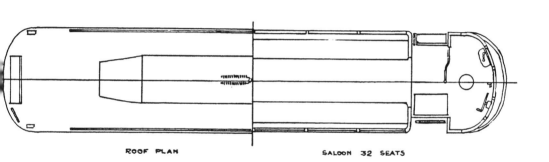

ROOF PLAN                    SALOON 32 SEATS

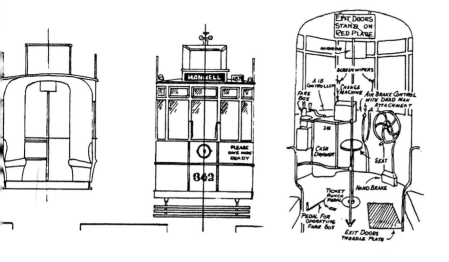

MANVELL   487

PLEASE HAVE FARE READY

342

EXIT DOORS STAND ON RED PLATE

MIRROR

SCREEN WIPERS

A.I.B. CONTROLLER

CHANGE MACHINE

AIR BRAKE CONTROL WITH DEAD MAN ATTACHMENT

FARE BOX

CASH DRAWER

SEAT

TICKET PUNCH PEDAL

HAND BRAKE

PEDAL FOR OPERATING FARE BOX

EXIT DOORS TREADLE PLATE

# LONDON UNITED TRAMWAYS

### ONE-MAN CAR    TYPE S2

342-344 CONVERTED 9/1925
ORIGINALLY    175, 178 & 275
WITHDRAWN 1928 SCRAPPED 1931
WORKED HANWELL-BRENTFORD LINE

COLOURS:      RED & WHITE
GOLD LINING & LETTERING

R. E. TUSTIN    5/56

0 1 2 3 4 5 6 7 8 9 10 11 12 13 14 15 16 17 18 19 20

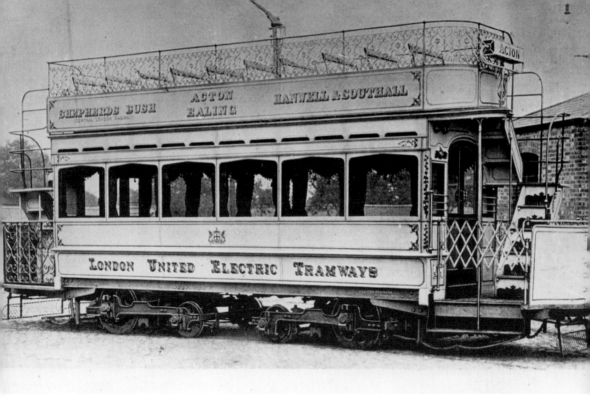

## TYPE X

115. The first hundred electric trams bought in 1900 were uncanopied, open top, eight wheel double deckers with double right angle stairs. They had Hurst Nelson bodywork, Peckham trucks, and BTH electrical equipment (see pictures 56 and 108) and they ran on all LUT routes. The next batch, numbered 101-150, as illustrated here, were basically similar, but from different manufacturers. They normally ran only on the Hanwell and Uxbridge services. (Tramway & Railway World)

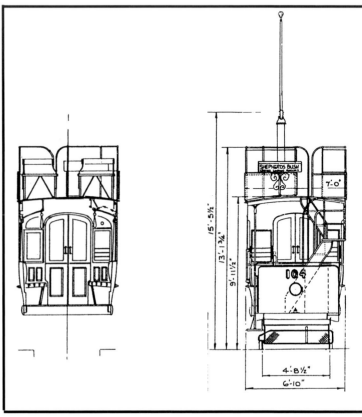

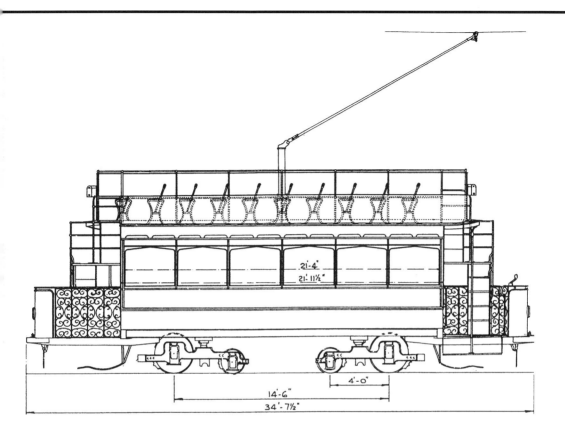

21'-4"
21'-11½"

4'-0"

14'-6"

34'-7½"

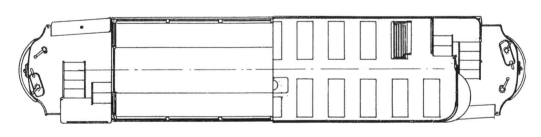

DRAWN BY:-TERRY RUSSELL, "CHACESIDE", ST.LEONARDS PARK, HORSHAM, W.SUSSEX. RH13 6EG.
SEND 4 FIRST CLASS STAMPS FOR COMPLETE LIST OF PUBLIC TRANSPORT DRAWINGS.

SCALE
FEET  0  1  2  3  4  5  6  7  8  9  10  11  12

LONDON UNITED TRAMWAYS
OPEN TOP 8 WHEEL CAR

BUILT: MILNES 1901
TYPE: X. FLEET No 101-150

SCALE 4   MM = 1 FOOT

DRAWING No  TC596

# TYPE U

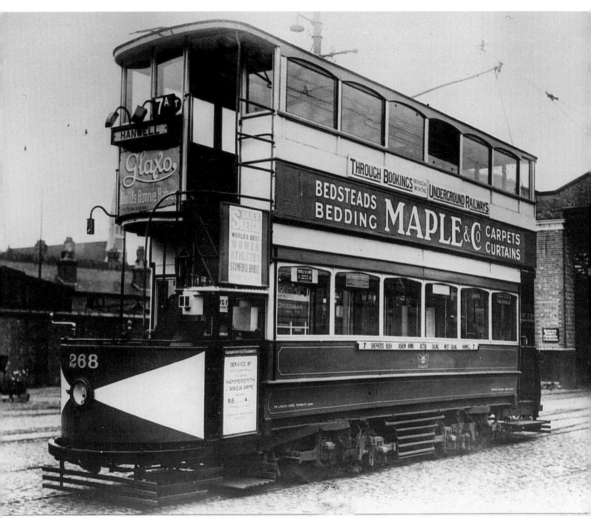

116. The next 150 trams, numbered 151-300, were almost identical with 101-150 for the bodywork and electrical equipment, but had Brill 22E bogies instead of McGuire trucks. Twenty-five of the bodies were built by the British Electric Car Company and 125 by Milnes. In 1910-11 covered tops were fitted to 66 cars of the 1-100 type, and to 35 cars of the 151-300 type, as illustrated here by car 268 in the forecourt of Hanwell Depot. When type codes were allocated in 1913-14, cars 1-100 became type Z with open tops and type Y with covered tops. Cars 101-150 became type X (none were ever top covered), and cars 151-300 became type W with open tops and type U with covered tops. A few of types U or W were later rebuilt as U2, UX, or WT, but did not run on Uxbridge Road. (Real Photographs)

# TYPE T

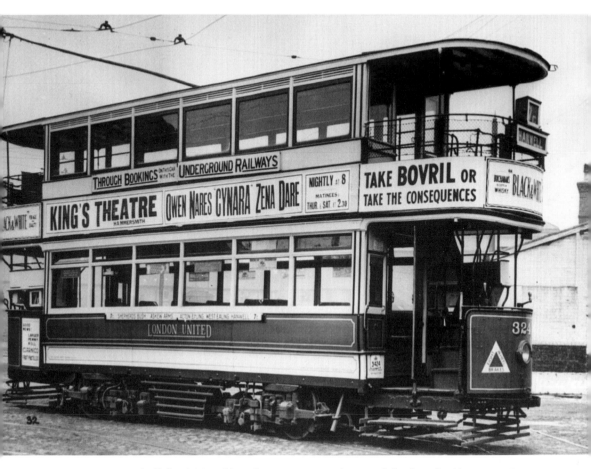

117. Cars 301-340 were built in 1906 and later became type T. They are fully described in companion volume *Kingston and Wimbledon Tramways*. Bodies were built by the UEC Company of Preston, bogies were by Brill and electrical equipment by Westinghouse. After an initial spell in the Kingston area, most spent their lives on the Uxbridge Road. Originally their destination boxes were higher up, but these were lowered when route number boxes were added. Here we have a splendid view of car 324 after overhaul in about 1925.   (Real Photographs)

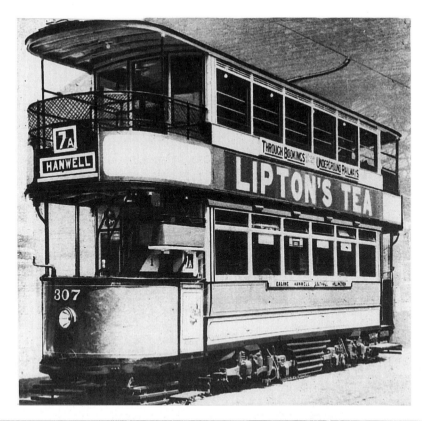

**TYPE UCC**

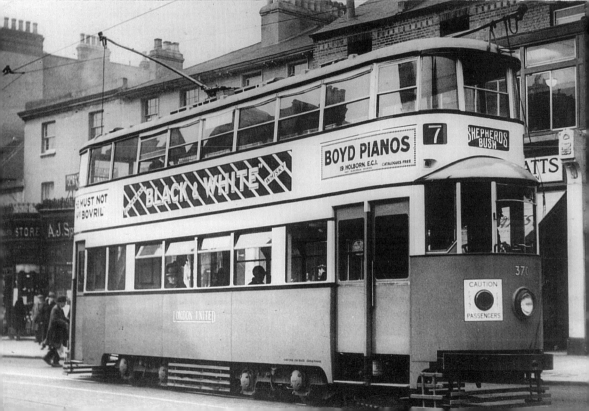

118. Only one of the T type, car 307, had destination and number boxes lowered still further in 1925. The seating on both decks was also improved. (Tramway & Railway World)

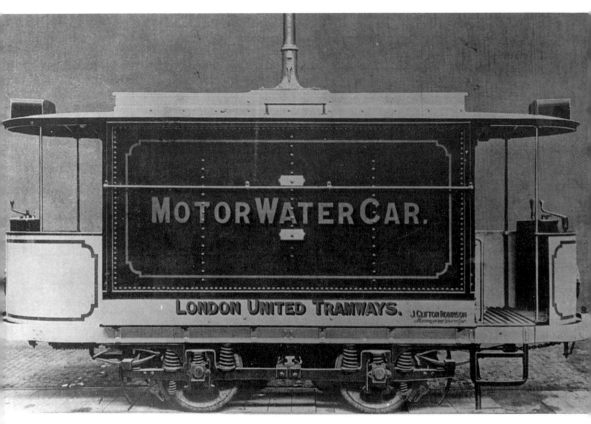

119. We come to the well known Feltham, or UCC type, of which 46, numbered 351-396, were built in 1930-31 by the Union Construction Co Ltd, a subsidiary of the UndergrounD group, at Feltham in Middlesex. A further 54 of identical design (described in *Edgware and Willesden Tramways*), except for different electrical equipment and the fitting of conduit plough carriers, were built for the Metropolitan Electric Tramways. Car 370 here is probably in Ealing Broadway. (John Gillham Coll.)

120. There were also six stores or works cars, numbered 001-006, including this water car, useful for spraying the track on a hot day to keep the dust down. See also picture 66. (John Gillham Coll.)

# MP Middleton Press

**Easebourne Lane, Midhurst, West Sussex. GU29 9AZ Tel: 01730 813169  Fax: 01730 812601**
*If books are not available from your local transport stockist, order direct with cheque, Visa or Mastercard, post free UK.*

## BRANCH LINES
Branch Line to Allhallows
Branch Lines to Alton
Branch Lines around Ascot
Branch Line to Ashburton
Branch Lines around Bodmin
Branch Line to Bude
Branch Lines around Canterbury
Branch Line to Cheddar
Branch Lines around Cromer
Branch Lines to East Grinstead
Branch Lines to Effingham Junction
Branch Line to Fairford
Branch Line to Hawkhurst
Branch Line to Hayling
Branch Lines to Horsham
Branch Line to Ilfracombe
Branch Line to Kingswear
Branch Lines to Launceston & Princetown
Branch Lines to Longmoor
Branch Line to Looe
Branch Line to Lyme Regis
Branch Lines around March
Branch Lines around Midhurst
Branch Line to Minehead
Branch Line to Moretonhampstead
Branch Lines to Newport (IOW)
Branch Line to Padstow
Branch Lines around Plymouth
Branch Line to Selsey
Branch Lines around Sheerness
Branch Line to Tenterden
Branch Lines to Torrington
Branch Lines to Tunbridge Wells
Branch Line to Upwell
Branch Lines around Weymouth
Branch Lines around Wimborne
Branch Lines around Wisbech

## NARROW GAUGE BRANCH LINES
Branch Line to Lynton
Branch Lines around Portmadoc 1923-46
Branch Lines around Porthmadog 1954-94
Branch Line to Southwold
Two-Foot Gauge Survivors

## SOUTH COAST RAILWAYS
Ashford to Dover
Brighton to Eastbourne
Chichester to Portsmouth
Dover to Ramsgate
Hastings to Ashford
Portsmouth to Southampton
Ryde to Ventnor
Southampton to Bournemouth
Worthing to Chichester

## SOUTHERN MAIN LINES
Bromley South to Rochester
Charing Cross to Orpington
Crawley to Littlehampton
Dartford to Sittingbourne
East Croydon to Three Bridges
Epsom to Horsham
Exeter to Barnstaple
Exeter to Tavistock
Faversham to Dover
Haywards Heath to Seaford
London Bridge to East Croydon
Orpington to Tonbridge
Swanley to Ashford
Tavistock to Plymouth

Victoria to East Croydon
Waterloo to Windsor
Waterloo to Woking
Woking to Portsmouth
Woking to Southampton
Yeovil to Exeter

## EASTERN MAIN LINES
Fenchurch Street to Barking

## COUNTRY RAILWAY ROUTES
Andover to Southampton
Bournemouth to Evercreech Jn.
Burnham to Evercreech Junction
Croydon to East Grinstead
Didcot to Winchester
Fareham to Salisbury
Frome to Bristol
Guildford to Redhill
Porthmadog to Blaenau
Reading to Basingstoke
Reading to Guildford
Redhill to Ashford
Salisbury to Westbury
Stratford Upon Avon to Cheltenham
Strood to Paddock Wood
Taunton to Barnstaple
Wenford Bridge to Fowey
Westbury to Bath
Woking to Alton
Yeovil to Dorchester

## GREAT RAILWAY ERAS
Ashford from Steam to Eurostar
Clapham Junction 50 years of change
Festiniog in the Fifties
Festiniog in the Sixties
Isle of Wight Lines 50 years of change
Railways to Victory 1944-46

## LONDON SUBURBAN RAILWAYS
Caterham and Tattenham Corner
Charing Cross to Dartford
Clapham Jn. to Beckenham Jn.
Crystal Palace and Catford Loop
East London Line
Finsbury Park to Alexandra Palace
Holborn Viaduct to Lewisham
Kingston and Hounslow Loops
Lewisham to Dartford
Lines around Wimbledon
London Bridge to Addiscombe
North London Line
South London Line
West Croydon to Epsom
West London Line
Willesden Junction to Richmond
Wimbledon to Epsom

## STEAM PHOTOGRAPHERS
O.J.Morris's Southern Railways 1919-59

## STEAMING THROUGH
Steaming through Cornwall
Steaming through the Isle of Wight
Steaming through Kent
Steaming through West Hants
Steaming through West Sussex

## TRAMWAY CLASSICS
Aldgate & Stepney Tramways
Barnet & Finchley Tramways

Bath Tramways
Bournemouth & Poole Tramways
Brighton's Tramways
Bristol's Tramways
Camberwell & W.Norwood Tramways
Clapham & Streatham Tramways
Dover's Tramways
East Ham & West Ham Tramways
Edgware and Willesden Tramways
Eltham & Woolwich Tramways
Embankment & Waterloo Tramways
Enfield & Wood Green Tramways
Exeter & Taunton Tramways
Gosport & Horndean Tramways
Greenwich & Dartford Tramways
Hampstead & Highgate Tramways
Hastings Tramways
Holborn & Finsbury Tramways
Ilford & Barking Tramways
Kingston & Wimbledon Tramways
Lewisham & Catford Tramways
Liverpool Tramways 1. Eastern Routes
Liverpool Tramways 2. Southern Routes
Maidstone & Chatham Tramways
North Kent Tramways
Portsmouth's Tramways
Reading Tramways
Seaton & Eastbourne Tramways
Southampton Tramways
Southend-on-sea Tramways
Southwark & Deptford Tramways
Stamford Hill Tramways
Thanet's Tramways
Victoria & Lambeth Tramways
Waltham Cross & Edmonton Tramways
Walthamstow & Leyton Tramways
Wandsworth & Battersea Tramways

## TROLLEYBUS CLASSICS
Croydon Trolleybuses
Bournemouth Trolleybuses
Maidstone Trolleybuses
Reading Trolleybuses
Woolwich & Dartford Trolleybuses

## WATERWAY ALBUMS
Kent and East Sussex Waterways
London's Lost Route to the Sea
London to Portsmouth Waterway
Surrey Waterways
West Sussex Waterways

## MILITARY BOOKS and VIDEO
Battle over Portsmouth
Battle over Sussex 1940
Blitz over Sussex 1941-42
Bombers over Sussex 1943-45
Bognor at War
Military Defence of West Sussex
Secret Sussex Resistance
Sussex Home Guard
War on the Line
War on the Line VIDEO

## OTHER BOOKS and VIDEO
Betwixt Petersfield & Midhurst
Brickmaking in Sussex
Changing Midhurst
Garraway Father & Son
Index to all Stations
South Eastern & Chatham Railways
London Chatham & Dover Railway